Viewing Food Through the Lens of Nourishment

Viewing Food Through the Lens of Nourishment

A Comprehensive Guide to Mastering Healthy Cooking

Dr. *A*. Romani

LEAFY PEN

(Leafy Pen™)

Leafy Pen / Leafy Pen™

Mt Prospect, Il USA
1-(888) 821-3271
www.LeafyPen.com

Published by **Dr. *A*. Romani** / Leafy Pen (Leafy Pen™)
ISBN 979-8-9990430-0-9

Viewing Food Through the Lens of Nourishment: A Comprehensive Guide to Healthy Cooking

DISCLAIMER: The information and/or statements presented herein have not been evaluated by the Food and Drug Administration and is not intended to diagnose, treat, cure or prevent any disease. The information in this book, other print types or digital (eBook) is just that... information, and is used for informational purposes only and is not intended to be a substitute for any medical diagnosis, advice or treatment. Your reliance on this information is to be solely at your own risk. Always seek out professional medical advice or treatment from a professional/Doctor.

ISBN: 979-8-9990430-0-9 (print, hardcover)
ISBN: 979-8-9990430-1-6 (eBook)

Library of Congress Control Number: 2025906415

BISAC: HEA013000. | HEA017000. | CKB039000.

Dedication

I truly dedicate this book to every beloved book reader all over the world. I couldn't have made this possible without such passionate readers. Thank you for your support, and continuing support.

Table of Contents

Introduction

Welcome to "*Viewing Food Through the Lens of Nourishment:* A Comprehensive Guide to Mastering Healthy Cooking." This book is designed to be your trusted companion on a transformative journey towards a healthier, more vibrant lifestyle through the power of nutritious and delicious cooking. In the pages that follow, you'll discover a wealth of knowledge, practical tips, and inspiring recipes that will revolutionize your approach to food and empower you to take control of your well-being through mindful, health-conscious culinary practices.

The journey to mastering healthy cooking is one of discovery, creativity, and personal growth. It's about more than just following recipes or counting calories; it's about developing a deep understanding of how food nourishes your body and impacts your overall health. As you progress through this book, you'll gain the confidence and skills needed to make informed choices about the ingredients you use, the cooking methods you employ, and the meals you create. You'll learn to view your kitchen as a place of innovation and experimentation, where you can craft meals that are not only good for you but also satisfying and enjoyable.

Throughout this guide, we'll explore the intricate relationship between food and health, delving into the science of nutrition while keeping things practical and accessible. You'll learn how to navigate the often-confusing world of dietary advice, understanding how to balance macronutrients and micronutrients to support your body's needs. We'll demystify food labels, explore the benefits of whole foods, and discuss how to make smart choices when shopping for ingredients.

But knowledge alone isn't enough to transform your cooking habits. That's why this book is packed with actionable advice, step-by-step techniques, and a wide variety of recipes designed to suit different tastes, dietary requirements, and skill levels. From quick and easy weeknight dinners to more elaborate dishes for special occasions, you'll find inspiration for every meal of the day. Each recipe is crafted not just for its nutritional profile, but also for its flavor and appeal, proving that healthy eating doesn't mean sacrificing taste or enjoyment.

As we embark on this culinary adventure together, remember that healthy cooking is a skill that can be learned and refined over time. It's a journey of continuous learning and adaptation. The goal of this book is not to prescribe a one-size-fits-all approach to eating, but rather to equip you with the knowledge and tools to make choices that align with your personal health goals and lifestyle. Whether you're looking to lose weight, manage a health condition, or simply feel more energized and vibrant, the principles and practices outlined in this guide will serve as a foundation for your success.

Embarking on Your Healthy Cooking Journey

The decision to embark on a healthy cooking journey is a powerful commitment to your well-being. It's a choice that goes beyond mere sustenance, embracing food as a source of nourishment, healing, and joy. As you begin this journey, it's important to recognize that transforming your cooking habits is a process that requires patience, persistence, and a willingness to learn. Like any worthwhile endeavor, mastering healthy cooking takes time and practice, but the rewards are immeasurable in terms of improved health, increased energy, and a deeper connection to the food you eat.

One of the first steps in your healthy cooking journey is to shift your perspective on food. Rather than viewing certain foods as "good" or "bad," start thinking about how different ingredients can contribute to your overall well-being. Whole, unprocessed foods should form the foundation of your diet, providing a rich array of nutrients that support your body's functions. Fresh fruits and vegetables, whole grains, lean proteins, and healthy fats are the building blocks of nutritious meals. As you become more familiar with these ingredients, you'll discover new flavors and textures that can make healthy eating an exciting culinary adventure.

Understanding the basics of nutrition is crucial as you begin your journey. You'll learn about the importance of balancing macronutrients (carbohydrates, proteins, and fats) and ensuring you get an adequate supply of micronutrients (vitamins and minerals). This knowledge will empower you to make informed decisions about the foods you choose and how you combine them to create balanced meals. Remember, healthy eating isn't about deprivation or strict rules; it's about nourishing your body with a variety of nutrient-dense foods that support your health goals.

As you progress on your healthy cooking journey, you'll develop new skills and techniques that will make preparing nutritious meals easier and more enjoyable. You'll learn how to use herbs and spices to enhance flavor without relying on excessive salt or sugar. You'll discover cooking methods that preserve the nutritional value of ingredients while creating delicious dishes. And you'll gain confidence in adapting recipes to suit your tastes and dietary needs. These skills will not only improve your cooking but will also give you the flexibility to create healthy meals even when you're short on time or working with limited ingredients.

One of the most important aspects of your healthy cooking journey is developing a positive relationship with food. This means learning to enjoy the process of cooking, savoring your meals mindfully, and listening to your body's hunger and fullness cues. It also involves finding a balance that works for you, allowing for occasional indulgences without guilt. Remember, healthy eating is not about perfection; it's about making choices that nourish your body and soul most of the time.

As you embark on this journey, it's helpful to set realistic goals and celebrate your progress along the way. Start by making small, sustainable changes to your cooking habits. Perhaps you'll commit to trying one new vegetable each week or experimenting with a different whole grain. Maybe you'll focus on mastering a particular cooking technique or on reducing your reliance on processed foods. Whatever your starting point, remember that every healthy meal you prepare is a step in the right direction.

Throughout your journey, don't be afraid to experiment and make mistakes. Cooking is an art as much as it is a science, and some of the best culinary discoveries come from unexpected places. If a recipe doesn't turn out as planned, try to learn from the experience. What could you do differently next time? How might you adjust the flavors or cooking method to better suit your tastes? This spirit of curiosity and willingness to learn will serve you well as you continue to grow and evolve in your healthy cooking practices.

Remember that your healthy cooking journey is uniquely yours. While this book provides guidance and inspiration, it's up to you to find the approach that works best for your lifestyle, preferences, and health needs. Be patient with yourself as you learn and grow, and don't hesitate to seek support when you need it. Whether it's joining a cooking class, connecting with like-minded individuals online, or simply sharing your new recipes with friends and family, building a supportive community can help keep you motivated and inspired on your journey.

As you embark on this exciting adventure in healthy cooking, keep in mind that the benefits extend far beyond the kitchen. By nourishing your body with wholesome, nutritious foods, you're investing in your long-term health and well-being. You may find that you have more energy, better digestion, improved mood, and a greater sense of overall vitality. Moreover, the skills and knowledge you gain will empower you to take control of your health in a fundamental way, giving you the tools to adapt to changing needs and circumstances throughout your life.

So, take a deep breath, open your mind to new possibilities, and get ready to transform your relationship with food. Your healthy cooking journey starts now, and the pages that follow will guide you every step of the way. Remember, every great chef and home cook started as a beginner, and with dedication and practice, you too can master the art of healthy cooking. Let's begin this delicious adventure together!

What to Expect from This Book

"*Viewing Food Through the Lens of Nourishment: A Comprehensive Guide to Mastering Healthy Cooking*" is designed to be your go-to resource for all things related to nutritious and delicious cooking. This book is structured to take you on a logical journey, building your knowledge and skills progressively as you move through each chapter. Whether you're a complete novice in the kitchen or an experienced cook looking to make healthier choices, you'll find valuable information and practical advice that you can apply immediately to your cooking routine.

The book begins with a solid foundation in nutrition basics, helping you understand the role of various nutrients in your body and how to create balanced meals. You'll learn about macronutrients and micronutrients, how to read food labels, and how to make informed choices about the foods you eat. This knowledge will serve as the cornerstone for your healthy cooking journey, empowering you to make decisions that align with your health goals.

From there, we'll dive into the practical aspects of healthy cooking, starting with ingredient selection. You'll discover how to choose the freshest, most nutritious ingredients and how to stock your kitchen with healthy staples. We'll explore the benefits of whole foods, seasonal produce, and discuss the pros and cons of organic versus conventional options. This section will equip you with the knowledge to navigate grocery stores and farmers' markets with confidence, selecting ingredients that will form the basis of your healthy meals.

The book then moves on to essential cooking techniques that preserve nutrients and enhance flavor without relying on excessive fats or artificial additives. You'll learn methods such as steaming, roasting, grilling, and sautéing, understanding how each technique can be used to create delicious, health-promoting meals. We'll also cover meal planning and preparation strategies to help you maintain a healthy diet even with a busy lifestyle. You'll discover tips for efficient grocery shopping, batch cooking, and proper food storage that will save you time and reduce waste.

A significant portion of the book is dedicated to recipes, covering everything from energizing breakfasts to satisfying dinners and smart snacks. Each recipe is carefully crafted to be nutritionally balanced, flavorful, and achievable for home cooks. You'll find options suitable for various dietary needs, including plant-based, gluten-free, and low-sodium diets. These recipes are more than just instructions; they're designed to inspire creativity and confidence in the kitchen, encouraging you to experiment and adapt them to your tastes.

Beyond recipes, you'll find chapters dedicated to specific aspects of healthy cooking, such as enhancing flavor naturally with herbs and spices, cooking for special dietary needs, and practicing mindful eating. These sections provide deeper insights into how you can tailor your cooking to support specific health goals or dietary requirements. You'll learn how to create flavorful meals without relying on salt or sugar, how to adapt recipes for common food allergies or intolerances, and how to develop a more mindful approach to eating that may improve your overall relationship with food.

Throughout the book, you'll find practical tips and informative sidebars that provide additional context and guidance. These features are designed to make the information more accessible and easier to apply in your daily life. You'll also find suggestions for further reading and resources if you wish to delve deeper into specific topics.

One of the unique aspects of this book is its emphasis on sustainable cooking practices. You'll learn how to reduce food waste, make eco-friendly food choices, and select sustainable kitchen equipment.

This section reflects the growing understanding that our food choices impact not only our personal health but also the health of our planet.

The book concludes with a comprehensive appendix and glossary, providing quick reference guides for measurement conversions, cooking times for common ingredients, and definitions of culinary terms. These resources will prove invaluable as you continue to explore and experiment in the kitchen.

As you progress through the book, you'll notice that each chapter builds upon the knowledge and skills introduced in previous sections. This cumulative approach allows you to gradually expand your culinary repertoire and deepen your understanding of healthy cooking principles. By the time you reach the end of the book, you'll have a comprehensive toolkit for creating nutritious, delicious meals that support your health and well-being.

Remember, this book is not meant to be read passively. To get the most out of it, try to actively engage with the material. Experiment with the recipes, practice the techniques, and reflect on how the information applies to your personal health journey. Don't be afraid to make notes, highlight sections that resonate with you, or bookmark recipes you want to try. This book is a resource that you can return to again and again as you continue to grow and evolve in your healthy cooking journey.

Above all, "Viewing Food" is designed to inspire and empower you. It's not about prescribing a rigid set of rules, but rather about providing you with the knowledge and tools to make informed choices that work for you. As you explore the pages that follow, remember that healthy cooking is a skill that improves with practice. Be patient with yourself, celebrate your successes, and most importantly, enjoy the process of nourishing yourself and your loved ones with delicious, health-promoting meals.

Shifting Your Mindset: Food as Nourishment

One of the most crucial steps in your journey towards healthier cooking and eating is shifting your mindset about food. In our modern society, food is often viewed through various lenses - as a source of comfort, a social lubricant, a reward, or even as the enemy in our quest for health or weight management. While food can indeed serve many purposes in our lives, the fundamental shift we need to make is to view food primarily as nourishment for our bodies and minds. This perspective change is not about restriction or deprivation; rather, it's about understanding and appreciating the profound impact that food has on our overall well-being.

When you begin to see food as nourishment, you start to make choices based on how foods will fuel your body and support your health, rather than solely on taste or convenience. This doesn't mean that food can't or shouldn't be enjoyable - quite the opposite. When you choose foods that truly nourish you, you'll likely find that you feel better overall, which can lead to a greater appreciation and enjoyment of your meals. It's about finding the balance between pleasure and nutrition, understanding that these two aspects of eating are not mutually exclusive but can work in harmony to support a healthy lifestyle.

This shift in mindset involves developing a deeper understanding of how different foods affect your body. For example, when you eat a meal rich in whole grains, lean proteins, and vegetables, you're not just satisfying your hunger - you're providing your body with a complex array of nutrients that support everything from your energy levels to your immune system. On the other hand, when you consistently choose processed foods high in sugar and unhealthy fats, you may be compromising your health in both the short and long term. By viewing food through the lens of nourishment, you become more attuned to these effects and can make choices that align with your health goals.

Another important aspect of this mindset shift is moving away from the dichotomy of "good" and "bad" foods. While some foods are certainly more nutrient-dense than others, labeling foods as inherently good or bad can lead to an unhealthy relationship with eating. Instead, think about foods in terms of their nutritional value and how they make you feel. Some foods might be best enjoyed in moderation, while others can form the foundation of your daily diet. This nuanced approach allows for flexibility and enjoyment while still prioritizing overall health.

Shifting your mindset also involves reconnecting with your food in a more meaningful way. In our fast-paced world, it's easy to fall into the habit of mindless eating - consuming meals quickly without really thinking about what we're putting into our bodies. When you view food as nourishment, you're more likely to engage in mindful eating practices. This might involve taking the time to prepare meals from scratch, savoring the flavors and textures of your food, and paying attention to your body's hunger and fullness cues. These practices not only enhance your enjoyment of food but also help you make more conscious, health-promoting choices.

It's important to recognize that this shift in mindset is a process that takes time and patience. You may have deeply ingrained habits or beliefs about food that have been formed over many years. Be gentle with yourself as you work on changing these patterns. Start by making small, manageable changes - perhaps focusing on adding more vegetables to your meals or taking a few extra minutes to really enjoy your food without distractions. Over time, these small changes can lead to significant shifts in how you think about and interact with food.

As you work on viewing food as nourishment, you may find it helpful to educate yourself about the nutritional content of different foods. Understanding what nutrients your body needs and how different foods can provide these nutrients can be empowering. This knowledge allows you to make informed choices about what to eat, not based on external rules or fad diets, but on a genuine understanding of what your body needs to thrive.

Remember that nourishment goes beyond just the physical aspects of food. The social and emotional components of eating are also important for overall well-being. Sharing meals with loved ones, celebrating special occasions with traditional foods, or finding comfort in a favorite dish are all valid and important aspects of our relationship with food. The key is to find a balance where these experiences can coexist with a focus on nourishing your body.

As you progress through this book and continue on your healthy cooking journey, keep coming back to this fundamental idea of food as nourishment. Let it guide your choices in the grocery store, your experiments in the kitchen, and your approach to mealtimes. With practice, you'll find that this perspective becomes second nature, leading to a more positive and balanced relationship with food that supports your overall health and well-being.

Embracing food as nourishment is not about perfection or adhering to strict rules. It's about developing a deeper appreciation for the role that food plays in your life and health. It's about making choices that honor your body's needs while still allowing for enjoyment and flexibility. As you continue to explore healthy cooking, let this mindset be your guide, informing your decisions and inspiring you to create meals that are truly nourishing in every sense of the word.

Description

Elevate your culinary skills and revolutionize your approach to healthy eating with "*Viewing Food Through the Lens of Nourishment*: A Comprehensive Guide to Mastering Healthy Cooking." This book is your ultimate companion in the kitchen, designed to empower you with the knowledge and techniques needed to create delicious, nutritious meals that fuel your body and delight your taste buds. From understanding the fundamentals of nutrition to mastering advanced cooking techniques, this guide takes you on a culinary journey that will transform the way you approach food. You'll learn how to select the freshest ingredients, balance flavors, and create meals that are both satisfying and health-promoting. Whether you're looking to improve your overall well-being, manage your weight, or simply enjoy more vibrant and flavorful meals, "*Viewing Food Through the Lens of Nourishment*" provides you with the tools and inspiration to make healthy cooking a joyful and rewarding part of your daily routine. Get ready to discover a world of culinary possibilities that will nourish your body, mind, and soul.

Chapter 1: Understanding Nutrition Basics

Embarking on a journey towards healthier cooking and eating begins with a solid understanding of nutrition fundamentals. This chapter serves as the cornerstone of your culinary transformation, providing you with the essential knowledge to make informed decisions about the food you prepare and consume. By grasping these nutrition basics, you'll be better equipped to create meals that not only tantalize your taste buds but also nourish your body effectively.

Nutrition is the science that interprets the interaction of nutrients and other substances in food in relation to maintenance, growth, reproduction, health, and disease of an organism. It includes food intake, absorption, assimilation, biosynthesis, catabolism, and excretion. A proper understanding of nutrition can help you optimize your health, prevent chronic diseases, and enhance your overall well-being. As you delve into the world of healthy cooking, this foundational knowledge will empower you to make choices that align with your health goals and dietary needs.

Throughout this chapter, we'll explore the building blocks of nutrition, breaking down complex concepts into digestible information that you can readily apply to your cooking practices. From the role of macronutrients and micronutrients to the principles of creating a balanced diet, you'll gain insights that will transform the way you approach food preparation. We'll also delve into the concept of nutrient density, which is crucial for maximizing the nutritional value of your meals without compromising on flavor or satisfaction.

As we progress through each section, keep in mind that nutrition is not about restrictive diets or deprivation. Instead, it's about making informed choices that support your body's needs while still enjoying the pleasures of eating. The knowledge you gain here will serve as a compass, guiding you towards creating meals that are both delicious and nutritionally sound. Let's begin this enlightening journey into the world of nutrition, setting the stage for your success in mastering the art of healthy cooking.

Macronutrients: Carbohydrates, Proteins, and Fats

Macronutrients are the nutrients that your body requires in large amounts to function properly. They are the primary sources of energy and are essential for various bodily functions, including growth, metabolism, and tissue repair. The three main macronutrients are carbohydrates, proteins, and fats. Understanding the role of each macronutrient is crucial for creating balanced meals that meet your nutritional needs.

Carbohydrates are your body's primary source of energy. They are broken down into glucose, which fuels your brain, muscles, and other organs. Carbohydrates can be classified into two main categories: simple carbohydrates and complex carbohydrates. Simple carbohydrates, found in foods like fruits, milk, and table sugar, are quickly digested and can cause rapid spikes in blood sugar levels. Complex carbohydrates, found in whole grains, legumes, and vegetables, are digested more slowly, providing a steady release of energy and helping to maintain stable blood sugar levels. When cooking healthy meals, focus on incorporating complex carbohydrates, which also provide fiber, vitamins, and minerals.

Proteins are essential for building and repairing tissues, producing enzymes and hormones, and supporting immune function. They are made up of amino acids, often referred to as the building blocks of life. There are *20* different amino acids, nine of which are considered essential because your body cannot produce them on its own. These must be obtained through your diet. Protein sources can be categorized as complete or incomplete. Complete proteins, typically found in animal products like meat, fish, eggs, and dairy, contain all nine essential amino acids. Plant-based proteins, such as those found in legumes, nuts, and grains, are often incomplete but can be combined to provide all essential amino acids. When planning your meals, aim to include a variety of protein sources to ensure you're getting all the necessary amino acids.

Fats, contrary to popular misconception, are a vital part of a healthy diet. They provide energy, help absorb certain vitamins and are crucial for hormone production and cell membrane structure. However, not all fats are created equal. Unsaturated fats, found in foods like avocados, nuts, seeds, and olive oil, are considered heart-healthy and can help reduce inflammation in the body. Saturated fats, primarily found in animal products and some tropical oils, should be consumed in moderation as they can raise cholesterol levels when consumed in excess. Trans fats, often found in processed foods, are considered harmful and should be avoided. When cooking, opt for healthy fats like olive oil, avocado oil, or nut oils to enhance flavor and nutritional value.

Balancing these macronutrients in your meals is key to maintaining optimal health. While individual needs may vary based on factors such as age, sex, activity level, and health status, a general guideline for a balanced diet is to aim for *45-65%* of calories from carbohydrates, *10-35%* from protein, and *20-35%* from fats. However, these percentages can be adjusted based on your specific health goals and dietary preferences. For example, athletes may require a higher percentage of carbohydrates to fuel their intense physical activities, while someone following a ketogenic diet might consume a higher percentage of fats and lower percentage of carbohydrates.

When planning your meals, consider the macronutrient composition of different foods. For instance, a balanced meal might include a serving of lean protein (such as grilled chicken or tofu), a portion of complex carbohydrates (like brown rice or quinoa), and a source of healthy fats (such as avocado or olive oil-dressed salad). This combination ensures you're getting a mix of all three macronutrients, which can help keep you feeling satisfied and energized.

It's important to note that while counting macronutrients can be helpful for some individuals, it's not necessary for everyone. The key is to focus on consuming a variety of whole, nutrient-dense foods that provide a natural balance of macronutrients. As you become more familiar with the macronutrient content of different foods, you'll find it easier to create balanced meals intuitively.

In your journey towards healthier cooking, experiment with different combinations of macronutrients to find what works best for your body and lifestyle. Remember that the quality of the macronutrients is just as important as the quantity. Choose whole, minimally processed sources of carbohydrates, lean proteins, and healthy fats to maximize the nutritional value of your meals. By understanding and balancing macronutrients, you'll be well on your way to creating nourishing meals that support your overall health and well-being.

Micronutrients: Vitamins and Minerals

While macronutrients provide the bulk of your energy needs, micronutrients are equally crucial for maintaining optimal health. Micronutrients, as the name suggests, are nutrients required by the body in smaller amounts but are essential for various physiological functions. These include vitamins and minerals, which play vital roles in everything from bone health to immune function, energy production, and cellular repair. Understanding the importance of micronutrients and how to incorporate them into your cooking is key to creating truly nourishing meals.

Vitamins are organic compounds that your body needs to function properly. They are divided into two categories: fat-soluble vitamins (*A*, *D*, *E*, and *K*) and water-soluble vitamins (*B*-complex vitamins and vitamin *C*). Fat-soluble vitamins can be stored in the body's fatty tissues and liver, while water-soluble vitamins are not stored in large amounts and need to be replenished more frequently. Each vitamin has specific functions in the body. For example, vitamin *A* is crucial for vision and immune function, vitamin *C* is important for collagen production and acts as an antioxidant, and *B* vitamins play key roles in energy metabolism. When planning your meals, aim to include a variety of colorful fruits and vegetables, which are rich sources of many vitamins.

Minerals are inorganic elements that are essential for various bodily functions. They are categorized into macrominerals (needed in larger amounts) and trace minerals (needed in smaller amounts). Macrominerals include calcium, phosphorus, magnesium, sodium, potassium, chloride, and sulfur. Trace minerals include iron, manganese, copper, iodine, zinc, cobalt, fluoride, and selenium. Each mineral has specific roles in the body. For instance, calcium is crucial for bone health, iron is essential for oxygen transport in the blood, and zinc is important for immune function and wound healing. To ensure you're getting a wide range of minerals, incorporate a variety of whole grains, legumes, nuts, seeds, fruits, and vegetables into your cooking.

One of the challenges in nutrition is that many micronutrients work synergistically, meaning they need each other to function optimally. For example, vitamin *D* is necessary for calcium absorption, and vitamin *C* enhances iron absorption from plant sources. This interconnectedness highlights the importance of consuming a varied diet rather than relying on single nutrients or supplements. When planning your meals, think about combining foods that enhance each other's nutritional benefits. For instance, pairing iron-rich leafy greens with vitamin *C*-rich citrus fruits can improve iron absorption.

It's important to note that while micronutrient deficiencies can lead to various health problems, excessive intake of certain vitamins and minerals can also be harmful. This is particularly true for fat-soluble vitamins and certain minerals, which can accumulate in the body. For most people, a balanced diet that includes a variety of whole foods is sufficient to meet micronutrient needs. However, certain populations, such as pregnant women, older adults, or those with specific health conditions, may require additional supplementation under the guidance of a healthcare professional.

When it comes to cooking, certain preparation methods can affect the micronutrient content of foods. For example, water-soluble vitamins can be lost during boiling, while some minerals may be more bioavailable when foods are cooked. To maximize the micronutrient content of your meals, consider these cooking tips:

- Steam or lightly stir-fry vegetables to retain water-soluble vitamins
- Use the water from cooked vegetables in soups or sauces to capture any leached nutrients
- Include a mix of raw and cooked vegetables in your meals
- Choose whole grains over refined grains to retain more minerals
- Pair foods rich in fat-soluble vitamins with healthy fats to enhance absorption

Understanding micronutrients can also help you make informed decisions about food choices. For instance, if you're looking to boost your immune system, you might focus on foods rich in vitamins *C* and *D*, zinc, and selenium. If you're concerned about bone health, you might emphasize calcium-rich foods along with those high in vitamin *D* and vitamin *K*. By being mindful of the micronutrient content of different foods, you can create meals that not only taste great but also provide targeted nutritional benefits.

As you continue your journey in healthy cooking, pay attention to the variety of colors on your plate. Different colored fruits and vegetables often indicate different micronutrient profiles. For example, orange and yellow produce are often rich in beta-carotene (a precursor to vitamin *A*), while leafy greens are excellent sources of folate and minerals like iron and calcium. By "eating the rainbow," you're more likely to cover a wide range of micronutrients in your diet.

Remember, the goal is not to obsess over individual nutrients but to create a diverse and balanced diet that naturally provides a wide range of micronutrients. As you become more familiar with the micronutrient content of different foods, you'll find it easier to intuitively create meals that are not only delicious but also nutritionally complete. By prioritizing micronutrient-rich whole foods in your cooking, you're taking a significant step towards optimizing your health and well-being.

Creating a Balanced Diet

Creating a balanced diet is a fundamental aspect of healthy eating and cooking. A balanced diet provides your body with the right proportions of nutrients it needs to function optimally, maintain health, and prevent chronic diseases. It's not about strict limitations or depriving yourself of the foods you love, but rather about feeling great, having more energy, improving your health, and stabilizing your mood. Understanding how to create a balanced diet is crucial for anyone looking to improve their overall well-being through nutrition.

The concept of a balanced diet has evolved over the years, moving away from rigid food group recommendations to a more flexible approach that emphasizes overall dietary patterns. While individual nutritional needs can vary based on factors such as age, sex, activity level, and health status, there are some general principles that apply to most people. The key components of a balanced diet include:

- Adequate calories to maintain a healthy weight
- A variety of foods from all food groups
- Appropriate portions of each food group
- Sufficient intake of essential nutrients
- Limited consumption of foods high in added sugars, sodium, and unhealthy fats

One widely recognized model for creating a balanced diet is the MyPlate guide, developed by the U.S. Department of Agriculture. This visual representation suggests that a balanced meal should consist of approximately:

- Half the plate filled with fruits and vegetables
- One-quarter of the plate with whole grains
- One-quarter of the plate with lean protein
- A serving of dairy or a calcium-rich alternative

When planning your meals, focus on incorporating a variety of nutrient-dense foods. These are foods that provide substantial amounts of vitamins, minerals, and other nutrients with relatively few calories. Examples include:

- Colorful fruits and vegetables
- Whole grains like quinoa, brown rice, and oats
- Lean proteins such as fish, poultry, legumes, and tofu
- Healthy fats from sources like nuts, seeds, avocados, and olive oil
- Low-fat dairy or fortified plant-based alternatives

Portion control is another crucial aspect of creating a balanced diet. Even healthy foods, when consumed in excess, can lead to weight gain and nutritional imbalances. Learning to recognize appropriate portion sizes can help you maintain balance in your diet. Some strategies for portion control include:

- Using smaller plates to make portions appear larger
- Measuring foods until you become familiar with appropriate serving sizes
- Filling half your plate with vegetables before adding other components
- Being mindful of calorie-dense foods like nuts, oils, and avocados
- Listening to your body's hunger and fullness cues

While creating a balanced diet, it's important to consider the concept of food synergy. This refers to the way different foods work together to provide greater health benefits than when consumed individually. For example, combining vitamin C-rich foods with iron-rich plant foods enhances iron absorption. Similarly, pairing whole grains with legumes creates a complete protein source. By understanding these synergistic relationships, you can create meals that are not only balanced but also optimized for nutrient absorption and utilization.

Hydration is often overlooked but is a crucial component of a balanced diet. Water plays a vital role in nearly every bodily function, from regulating body temperature to aiding in digestion and nutrient absorption. While individual water needs can vary, a general guideline is to aim for *8-10* cups of fluid per day, with water being the primary source. Other hydrating options include herbal teas, low-fat milk, and water-rich fruits and vegetables.

It's also important to address the role of treats and less nutritious foods in a balanced diet. While the focus should be on nutrient-dense whole foods, there's room for occasional indulgences. The key is moderation and mindfulness. Rather than labeling foods as "good" or "bad," consider how they fit into your overall dietary pattern. Enjoying a small dessert or a favorite snack from time to time can be part of a balanced approach to eating, as long as it doesn't displace too many nutrient-dense foods from your diet.

Creating a balanced diet is not a one-size-fits-all approach. It's about finding what works best for your body, lifestyle, and preferences. Some people may thrive on three larger meals a day, while others may prefer smaller, more frequent meals. Some may choose to include animal products, while others may follow a plant-based diet. The key is to ensure that your overall dietary pattern provides all the nutrients your body needs in appropriate amounts.

As you embark on your journey of healthy cooking, use these principles of a balanced diet as a guide. Experiment with different combinations of foods, try new recipes, and pay attention to how different meals make you feel. Over time, you'll develop an intuitive sense of what constitutes a balanced diet for you. Remember, the goal is not perfection but progress towards a sustainable, enjoyable, and nourishing way of eating that supports your overall health and well-being.

Understanding Nutrient Density

Nutrient density is a concept that lies at the heart of healthy eating and cooking. It refers to the amount of beneficial nutrients in a food in proportion to its energy content (calories) or weight. Foods that are nutrient-dense provide substantial amounts of vitamins, minerals, and other beneficial compounds relative to their caloric content. Understanding and prioritizing nutrient density in your cooking can help you maximize the nutritional value of your meals while managing calorie intake, leading to improved overall health and well-being.

The concept of nutrient density is particularly important in today's food environment, where many readily available foods are high in calories but low in essential nutrients. These foods, often referred to as "empty calories," can contribute to weight gain and nutritional deficiencies if they make up a large part of the diet. By focusing on nutrient-dense foods, you can ensure that every calorie you consume is working hard to nourish your body and support optimal function.

Nutrient-dense foods typically include:

- Vegetables, especially leafy greens and cruciferous vegetables
- Fruits, particularly berries and citrus fruits
- Whole grains like quinoa, oats, and brown rice
- Legumes such as lentils, beans, and chickpeas
- Nuts and seeds
- Fatty fish like salmon, mackerel, and sardines
- Lean meats and poultry
- Eggs
- Low-fat dairy or fortified plant-based alternatives

When considering nutrient density, it's important to look beyond just vitamins and minerals. Other beneficial compounds, such as antioxidants, phytochemicals, and fiber, also contribute to a food's nutrient density. For example, berries are not only rich in vitamins but also contain powerful antioxidants that can help protect against cellular damage. Similarly, whole grains provide not just vitamins and minerals but also fiber, which is crucial for digestive health and can help manage blood sugar levels.

Incorporating nutrient-dense foods into your cooking doesn't mean you have to sacrifice flavor or enjoyment. In fact, many nutrient-dense foods are naturally flavorful and can be prepared in delicious ways. Here are some strategies for increasing the nutrient density of your meals:

- Start with a base of leafy greens in salads and grain bowls
- Add a variety of colorful vegetables to stir-fries, soups, and stews
- Use whole grains instead of refined grains in recipes
- Incorporate nuts and seeds into baked goods, salads, and as snacks
- Choose lean proteins and prepare them using healthy cooking methods like grilling or baking
- Use herbs and spices to add flavor without extra calories
- Include a serving of fruit with meals or as a naturally sweet dessert

It's worth noting that while focusing on nutrient density is generally beneficial, it's not the only factor to consider in a healthy diet. Some foods that are not particularly nutrient-dense, such as olive oil, can still play an important role in a balanced diet due to their other health benefits. The key is to strike a balance, ensuring that the majority of your diet consists of nutrient-dense foods while allowing for moderate amounts of other foods that contribute to overall dietary enjoyment and satisfaction.

When shopping for ingredients, reading nutrition labels can help you identify nutrient-dense options. Look for foods that provide high percentages of daily values for vitamins and minerals relative to their calorie content. However, be aware that not all beneficial compounds (such as phytochemicals) are listed on nutrition labels, which is why it's important to focus on whole, minimally processed foods as much as possible.

Cooking methods can also affect the nutrient density of foods. Some nutrients, particularly water-soluble vitamins, can be lost during cooking processes that involve high heat or large amounts of water. To preserve nutrient density when cooking:

- Steam or lightly stir-fry vegetables instead of boiling

- If boiling, use the cooking water in soups or sauces to retain leached nutrients
- Avoid overcooking, as this can degrade heat-sensitive nutrients
- Include a mix of raw and cooked vegetables in your meals
- Use the peel of fruits and vegetables when appropriate, as many nutrients are concentrated in or just under the skin

As you become more familiar with the concept of nutrient density, you may find it helpful to think in terms of "nutrient bang for your calorie buck." This mindset can guide you towards making food choices that provide the most nutritional benefit. For example, when choosing between two snacks with similar calorie content, opt for the one that provides a wider range of essential nutrients.

Remember that nutrient density is just one aspect of a healthy diet. Enjoyment, cultural significance, and personal preferences also play important roles in sustainable eating habits. The goal is to create a dietary pattern that is rich in nutrient-dense foods while still being enjoyable and aligned with your lifestyle and values.

By prioritizing nutrient density in your cooking and meal planning, you're taking a powerful step towards optimizing your health. You'll likely find that as you incorporate more nutrient-dense foods into your diet, your palate will adapt, and you'll develop a greater appreciation for the natural flavors and textures of whole, nutritious foods. This shift may not only benefit your physical health but can also enhance your overall relationship with food, leading to a more satisfying and nourishing approach to healthier eating.

Chapter 2: Selecting Quality Ingredients

The foundation of healthy cooking lies in the quality of ingredients you choose. This chapter delves into the art and science of selecting the best ingredients for your culinary creations. By understanding how to choose high-quality, nutrient-dense foods, you'll be able to elevate your cooking and enhance the nutritional value of your meals. The journey to mastering healthy cooking begins at the source - with the ingredients you bring into your kitchen.

In the following sections, you'll explore the importance of whole foods, learn how to navigate the world of seasonal produce, understand the differences between organic and conventional options, and develop the crucial skill of reading and interpreting food labels. These skills will empower you to make informed decisions about the foods you purchase and prepare, ultimately contributing to your overall health and well-being.

Remember, the quality of your ingredients directly impacts the nutritional value and taste of your meals. By investing time in selecting the best possible ingredients, you're setting yourself up for success in the kitchen and taking a significant step towards a healthier lifestyle. Let's dive into the world of ingredient selection and discover how to build a foundation for delicious, nutritious cooking.

The Power of Whole Foods

Whole foods are the cornerstone of a healthy diet and should form the basis of your ingredient selection. These are foods that are minimally processed and free from additives or artificial substances. They include fruits, vegetables, whole grains, legumes, nuts, seeds, and lean meats. The power of whole foods lies in their nutrient density and the complex interplay of vitamins, minerals, fiber, and phytochemicals they contain.

When you prioritize whole foods in your cooking, you're providing your body with a wide array of nutrients in their most natural and bioavailable form. This means your body can more easily absorb and utilize these nutrients for optimal health. For instance, an apple contains not just vitamin C, but also fiber, antioxidants, and a variety of other beneficial compounds that work synergistically. This complex nutritional profile is often lost in processed foods derived from apples, such as apple juice or apple-flavored snacks.

Incorporating whole foods into your diet has been associated with numerous health benefits. Research has shown that diets rich in whole foods can help reduce the risk of chronic diseases such as heart disease, type *2* diabetes, and certain cancers[1]. Whole foods are typically lower in added sugars, unhealthy fats, and sodium compared to their processed counterparts, making them an excellent choice for maintaining a healthy weight and supporting overall well-being.

When selecting whole foods, aim for variety. Different colors in fruits and vegetables often indicate different nutrient profiles. For example, orange and yellow produce like carrots and sweet potatoes are rich in beta-carotene, while leafy greens are excellent sources of folate and vitamin *K*. By "eating the rainbow," you ensure a diverse intake of nutrients.

It's important to note that while whole foods should form the majority of your diet, this doesn't mean you need to completely eliminate all processed foods. The key is to find a balance and make informed choices. When you do opt for packaged or processed items, look for those with minimal ingredients, all of which you can recognize and pronounce.

To incorporate more whole foods into your cooking:

- Start by replacing refined grains with whole grains. For instance, use brown rice instead of white rice, or whole wheat pasta instead of regular pasta.
- Snack on fresh fruits, vegetables, and nuts instead of packaged snacks.
- Use whole food ingredients to make homemade versions of typically processed foods. For example, make your own tomato sauce using fresh tomatoes instead of buying jarred sauce.
- When buying meat, choose cuts that haven't been processed or had additives included.
- Experiment with new whole foods regularly to expand your palate and nutrient intake.

Remember, transitioning to a whole foods-based diet is a journey. Start by making small, sustainable changes and gradually increase the proportion of whole foods in your diet. As you become more comfortable with selecting and preparing whole foods, you'll likely find that your taste preferences shift, and you'll naturally gravitate towards these nutrient-dense options.

Choosing Seasonal Produce

Selecting seasonal produce is a key strategy in enhancing the quality of your ingredients while supporting sustainable eating practices. Seasonal fruits and vegetables are typically harvested at their peak ripeness, which means they're not only bursting with flavor but also at their nutritional zenith. Understanding and embracing seasonality in your ingredient selection can significantly elevate your cooking while providing numerous benefits for your health, wallet, and the environment.

When produce is in season, it's generally more abundant, which often translates to lower prices at the market. This economic benefit allows you to purchase a wider variety of fruits and vegetables, encouraging dietary diversity. Moreover, seasonal produce often travels shorter distances from farm to table, reducing transportation costs and environmental impact. This shorter journey also means that the produce is fresher when it reaches you, retaining more of its nutritional value.

From a nutritional standpoint, seasonal eating aligns with nature's rhythms and our body's changing needs. For instance, many summer fruits are high in water content, helping to keep us hydrated during hot months. Winter vegetables like squashes and root vegetables are often rich in vitamins and minerals that support immune function during cold and flu season. By following nature's lead, you're providing your body with a natural variety of nutrients throughout the year.

To effectively incorporate seasonal produce into your cooking:

- Familiarize yourself with what's in season in your local area. This can vary depending on your geographical location and climate.
- Visit farmers' markets or join a Community Supported Agriculture (CSA) program to access fresh, local, seasonal produce.
- Be flexible with your meal planning. Instead of rigidly sticking to recipes, learn to substitute ingredients based on what's seasonally available.
- Learn preservation techniques like freezing, canning, or fermenting to extend the life of seasonal produce.
- Experiment with new fruits and vegetables as they come into season. This is a great way to expand your culinary repertoire and nutrient intake.

It's worth noting that while eating seasonally is beneficial, it doesn't mean you should completely avoid out-of-season produce. In many cases, frozen fruits and vegetables can be excellent alternatives when fresh, seasonal options aren't available. Frozen produce is typically harvested at peak ripeness and flash-frozen, locking in nutrients. This makes them a nutritious choice year-round, especially for items with short growing seasons.

When selecting seasonal produce, use your senses. Look for vibrant colors, firm textures, and fresh aromas. Avoid produce with blemishes, bruises, or signs of decay. Don't be afraid to ask vendors at farmers' markets about their produce - they're often passionate about their products and can provide valuable information about selection, storage, and preparation.

Remember, the goal is not perfection but progress. Even incorporating a few seasonal items into your regular shopping can make a difference. As you become more attuned to the rhythm of seasonal eating, you'll likely find yourself naturally gravitating towards this approach, enjoying the varied flavors and nutritional benefits that each season brings to your table.

Organic vs. Conventional: Making Informed Choices

The debate between organic and conventional produce is a complex one, with passionate advocates on both sides. As a health-conscious cook, it's important to understand the differences between these two categories and make informed decisions based on your personal health goals, budget, and values. This section will explore the key distinctions between organic and conventional produce, the potential benefits and drawbacks of each, and provide guidance on how to navigate these choices in your ingredient selection process.

Organic produce is grown without the use of synthetic pesticides, herbicides, or fertilizers. Instead, organic farmers rely on natural pest control methods and compost or manure for soil enrichment. Organic farming practices also prohibit the use of genetically modified organisms (GMOs) and growth hormones. On the other hand, conventional farming may use synthetic chemicals to control pests and weeds, as well as fertilizers to enhance soil productivity.

One of the primary arguments in favor of organic produce is the reduced exposure to pesticide residues. A study published in the journal Environmental Health Perspectives found that consuming organic produce can significantly reduce the levels of pesticide metabolites in the body[2]. This can be particularly important for certain populations, such as pregnant women and young children, who may be more susceptible to the potential effects of pesticide exposure.

However, it's important to note that both organic and conventional produce must meet safety standards set by regulatory bodies. The presence of pesticide residues on conventional produce is typically well below the established safe limits. Moreover, thorough washing of produce can help reduce surface residues, regardless of whether it's organic or conventional.

When it comes to nutritional content, the differences between organic and conventional produce are less clear-cut. While some studies have found slightly higher levels of certain nutrients in organic produce, the overall consensus is that the nutritional differences are minimal. The nutrient content of produce is influenced by many factors, including soil quality, climate, and the specific variety of the plant, rather than just whether it's grown organically or conventionally.

Environmental considerations often play a role in the organic vs. conventional debate. Organic farming practices are generally considered more environmentally friendly, promoting biodiversity and soil health. However, conventional farming can be more efficient in terms of land use, potentially allowing for higher yields on less land.

Cost is another factor to consider. Organic produce is often more expensive due to higher production costs and lower yields. This price difference can be a significant barrier for many consumers. If budget is a concern, it's worth noting that the nutritional benefits of eating a variety of fruits and vegetables, whether organic or conventional, far outweigh the potential risks of pesticide exposure from conventional produce.

To make informed choices between organic and conventional produce:

- Consider prioritizing organic for produce known to have higher pesticide residues, often referred to as the "Dirty Dozen." These typically include strawberries, spinach, kale, nectarines, and apples.
- For produce with lower pesticide residues, often called the "Clean Fifteen" (including avocados, sweet corn, pineapples, onions, and papayas), conventional options may be a cost-effective choice.

- Look for local produce, whether organic or conventional. Local farms often use fewer preservatives and may have more sustainable practices, even if not certified organic.
- Consider your personal health concerns. If you have specific health issues or are in a sensitive population group, consult with a healthcare provider about whether prioritizing organic produce would be beneficial.
- Remember that frozen or canned produce (without added sugars or sodium) can be nutritious and cost-effective alternatives, especially when fresh options are limited or expensive.

Ultimately, the choice between organic and conventional produce is a personal one that depends on various factors including health concerns, environmental values, and budget constraints. The most important thing is to consume a variety of fruits and vegetables, regardless of how they're grown. Both organic and conventional produce can be part of a healthy diet, and the benefits of eating plenty of fruits and vegetables far outweigh any potential risks associated with either farming method.

Reading and Understanding Food Labels

In today's complex food landscape, the ability to read and understand food labels is a crucial skill for making informed decisions about the ingredients you bring into your kitchen. Food labels provide a wealth of information about the nutritional content, ingredients, and production methods of packaged foods. By mastering the art of label reading, you can ensure that you're selecting products that align with your health goals and dietary preferences.

The Nutrition Facts panel is a key component of food labels, providing detailed information about the nutritional content of the product. Here's how to navigate this information effectively:

- Serving Size: Always check the serving size first. All the nutritional information on the label is based on this amount, which may be different from what you actually consume.
- Calories: This tells you how much energy you'll get from one serving of the food.
- Nutrients: The label lists key nutrients, including total fat, saturated fat, trans fat, cholesterol, sodium, total carbohydrates, dietary fiber, sugars, and protein. Pay particular attention to

saturated fat, added sugars, and sodium, as excessive intake of these has been linked to various health issues.

- Percent Daily Value (%DV): This shows how much of a nutrient in a serving of the food contributes to a total daily diet, based on a *2,000*-calorie diet. As a general guide, *5%* DV or less is considered low, while *20%* DV or more is high.

Beyond the Nutrition Facts panel, the ingredients list is another crucial component of food labels. Ingredients are listed in descending order by weight, meaning the first ingredient makes up the largest proportion of the product. When selecting packaged foods, look for products where whole food ingredients are listed first. Be wary of long ingredient lists with many unfamiliar or unpronounceable items, as these often indicate highly processed foods.

It's also important to be aware of common marketing terms and what they actually mean:

- "Natural" or "All Natural": This term is not strictly regulated and doesn't necessarily mean the product is healthier or free from artificial ingredients.
- "Organic": Products labeled "*100%* Organic" must contain only organically produced ingredients. Products labeled "Organic" must contain at least *95%* organic ingredients.
- "Low Fat" or "Reduced Fat": These products must meet specific criteria for fat content, but they may compensate by adding more sugar or sodium.
- "No Added Sugar": While this means no sugar has been added during processing, the product may still contain naturally occurring sugars.
- "Whole Grain": Look for "*100%* Whole Grain" to ensure all grains in the product are whole. "Made with Whole Grains" can mean only a small portion of the grains are whole.

When it comes to meat and poultry labels, terms like "Free Range," "Grass-Fed," and "Hormone-Free" have specific meanings defined by regulatory bodies. For example, "Grass-Fed" beef comes from cattle that have been fed only grass and forage throughout their lives, except for milk consumed prior to weaning. However, it's worth noting that this doesn't necessarily mean the animals had access to pasture.

For seafood, look for labels indicating sustainable sourcing, such as those certified by the Marine Stewardship Council (MSC) or the Aquaculture Stewardship Council (ASC). These certifications ensure that the seafood comes from well-managed fisheries or farms that minimize environmental impact.

When selecting packaged foods, a good rule of thumb is to choose products with shorter ingredient lists, focusing on those where you recognize most, if not all, of the ingredients. This often indicates a less processed product. However, don't be put off by scientific-sounding names for vitamins or minerals - for example, "ascorbic acid" is simply vitamin *C*.

Remember, while food labels provide valuable information, they should be considered in the context of your overall diet. No single food makes or breaks a healthy diet - it's the overall pattern of eating that matters most. Use label reading as a tool to make informed choices, but don't let it become an obsession that takes the joy out of eating.

By honing your label-reading skills, you'll be better equipped to select high-quality ingredients that align with your health goals and culinary preferences. This knowledge empowers you to make informed decisions in the grocery store, setting the stage for healthier, more nutritious cooking at home.

Chapter 3: Stocking Your Healthy Kitchen

A well-stocked kitchen is the foundation of healthy cooking. When you have the right ingredients and tools at your fingertips, preparing nutritious meals becomes effortless and enjoyable. This chapter will guide you through the essentials of stocking your kitchen for optimal health and culinary success. You'll learn about must-have pantry staples, fridge and freezer essentials, necessary cooking tools and equipment, and healthy ingredient substitutions that can elevate your cooking to new heights of nutrition and flavor.

By the end of this chapter, you'll have a comprehensive understanding of how to transform your kitchen into a haven for healthy cooking. You'll be equipped with the knowledge to make smart choices when shopping for ingredients and tools, ensuring that your kitchen is always ready to support your healthy lifestyle. Whether you're a seasoned cook or just starting your culinary journey, these insights will help you create a kitchen environment that inspires and facilitates nutritious meal preparation.

Essential Pantry Staples

A well-stocked pantry is the backbone of a healthy kitchen. It provides you with the foundation for countless nutritious meals and ensures that you always have the basics on hand to whip up a wholesome dish, even when fresh ingredients are scarce. When building your healthy pantry, focus on versatile, nutrient-dense items that have a long shelf life and can be used in a variety of recipes.

Whole grains should be a cornerstone of your pantry. These fiber-rich foods provide sustained energy and are packed with essential nutrients. Stock up on items like brown rice, quinoa, oats, and whole wheat pasta. These grains can serve as the base for many meals, from hearty breakfast bowls to satisfying dinner sides. Whole grain flours, such as whole wheat or almond flour, are also excellent to have on hand for baking healthier versions of your favorite treats.

Legumes are another pantry essential that offer a wealth of nutritional benefits. Dried or canned beans, lentils, and chickpeas are excellent sources of plant-based protein and fiber. They're incredibly versatile and can be used in soups, stews, salads, and even as meat substitutes in many dishes. Keep a variety on hand to add substance and nutrition to your meals. When opting for canned legumes, choose low-sodium options and rinse them before use to reduce sodium content further.

Nuts and seeds are nutritional powerhouses that deserve a place in your pantry. Almonds, walnuts, chia seeds, and flax seeds are rich in healthy fats, protein, and various micronutrients. They make excellent snacks on their own and can be used to add crunch and nutrition to salads, yogurt, and baked goods. Store them in airtight containers in a cool, dark place to maintain their freshness and prevent rancidity.

Healthy oils are essential for cooking and dressing your dishes. Extra virgin olive oil is a staple in Mediterranean cuisine and is known for its heart-healthy properties. Avocado oil is another excellent choice, with a high smoke point that makes it suitable for high-heat cooking. Coconut oil can be used in both sweet and savory dishes and offers unique health benefits. Having a variety of oils allows you to choose the best option for different cooking methods and flavor profiles.

Vinegars and condiments add flavor and depth to your cooking without relying on excessive salt or sugar. Stock your pantry with apple cider vinegar, balsamic vinegar, and rice vinegar for dressings and marinades. Mustard, hot sauce, and tamari (a gluten-free alternative to soy sauce) are versatile condiments that can elevate the taste of many dishes. Look for versions with minimal added sugars and preservatives.

Canned tomatoes and tomato paste are incredibly useful for creating quick sauces and adding depth to soups and stews. Choose varieties with no added salt or sugar to control the sodium and sugar content of your dishes. Similarly, low-sodium broths or bouillon cubes can serve as a base for soups or add flavor to grains and vegetables.

Dried herbs and spices are essential for adding flavor to your cooking without relying on salt or unhealthy additives. Build a collection of versatile spices like cumin, paprika, turmeric, and cinnamon. Dried herbs such as oregano, thyme, and basil can instantly elevate the taste of your dishes. Remember that spices lose their potency over time, so it's best to buy them in small quantities and replace them regularly.

Natural sweeteners like pure maple syrup, honey, and dates can be used in moderation to add sweetness to your cooking and baking. These options provide more nutrients and complexity of flavor compared to refined sugar. However, it's important to use them judiciously, as they still contribute to overall sugar intake.

Lastly, don't forget to stock some healthy convenience items. Canned fish like sardines or wild-caught salmon provide a quick source of protein and omega-3 fatty acids. Whole grain crackers, unsweetened dried fruits, and low-sodium jerky can serve as nutritious snacks or ingredients in more complex recipes.

By thoughtfully stocking your pantry with these essentials, you'll always be prepared to create healthy, delicious meals. Remember to rotate your pantry items regularly, using older products first and replenishing as needed. With these staples on hand, you'll find it easier to resist the temptation of unhealthy convenience foods and stay committed to your healthy cooking journey.

Fridge and Freezer Must-Haves

While a well-stocked pantry forms the foundation of a healthy kitchen, your refrigerator and freezer play equally crucial roles in supporting your nutritious cooking endeavors. These cold storage spaces are where you'll keep fresh produce, lean proteins, and other perishable items that are essential for creating balanced, wholesome meals. By strategically stocking your fridge and freezer, you'll ensure that you always have access to a variety of nutritious ingredients, even on busy days when you can't make it to the grocery store.

Let's start with the refrigerator. Fresh vegetables should be a priority in your fridge. Leafy greens like spinach, kale, and mixed salad greens are versatile and packed with nutrients. They can be used in salads, smoothies, or sautéed as a side dish. Cruciferous vegetables such as broccoli, cauliflower, and Brussels sprouts are excellent sources of fiber and antioxidants. Bell peppers, carrots, and celery are great for snacking and adding crunch to your meals. Remember to store your vegetables properly to maximize their shelf life. Most vegetables do best in the crisper drawer, where humidity levels can be controlled.

Fruits are another essential category for your fridge. While many fruits can be stored at room temperature, keeping them in the fridge can extend their freshness. Berries, grapes, and cut melons should always be refrigerated. Apples, pears, and citrus fruits can be kept in the fridge or at room temperature, depending on how quickly you plan to consume them. Having a variety of fruits on hand makes it easy to add natural sweetness and vital nutrients to your diet.

Lean proteins are a crucial component of a healthy diet, and your fridge is the perfect place to store them. Skinless chicken breasts, lean cuts of beef or pork, and fish fillets are excellent sources of protein that can be quickly prepared for meals. Eggs are another versatile protein source that can be used in countless ways. For plant-based options, consider keeping tofu or tempeh in your fridge. These soy-based proteins can be marinated and prepared in various ways to suit different recipes.

Dairy and dairy alternatives deserve a place in your fridge as well. If you consume dairy, opt for low-fat milk, yogurt, and cheese. Greek yogurt is particularly versatile, serving as a high-protein snack or a base for dips and dressings. For those who prefer non-dairy options, keep a variety of plant-based milks like almond, soy, or oat milk on hand. Many of these alternatives are fortified with calcium and vitamin *D*, making them nutritionally comparable to dairy milk.

Condiments and flavor enhancers are essential for bringing your dishes to life. Keep a selection of mustards, hot sauces, and pesto's in your fridge. These can add instant flavor to your meals without relying on excessive salt or sugar. Fresh herbs like cilantro, parsley, and basil can be stored in the fridge and used to add brightness to your cooking. Lemon and lime juice are also great to have on hand for adding acidity to dishes or dressings.

Now, let's turn our attention to the freezer. This often-underutilized space can be a treasure trove of healthy ingredients that are ready at a moment's notice. Frozen vegetables are an excellent option for busy cooks. They're picked at peak ripeness and flash-frozen, often retaining more nutrients than their fresh counterparts that have been transported long distances. Stock up on frozen spinach, peas, broccoli, and mixed vegetable blends. These can be quickly added to soups, stir-fries, or side dishes.

Frozen fruits are another freezer staple. Berries, mango chunks, and peach slices are perfect for smoothies or as toppings for yogurt and oatmeal. They can also be thawed and used in baking or as a naturally sweet dessert option. By keeping a variety of frozen fruits on hand, you'll always have access to nutritious, flavorful ingredients, even when fresh fruits are out of season.

Lean proteins can also be stored in the freezer for longer-term storage. Individually wrapped chicken breasts, fish fillets, or lean cuts of meat can be thawed as needed for meals. Ground turkey or lean beef can be portioned and frozen for easy use in recipes. For plant-based options, frozen edamame is a great source of protein that can be quickly added to meals.

Whole grains and bread products can be kept fresh in the freezer. Whole grain bread, tortillas, and even cooked grains like quinoa or brown rice can be frozen in portion-sized containers or bags. This allows you to always have healthy carbohydrate options available without worrying about spoilage.

Lastly, consider preparing and freezing some healthy convenience foods. Homemade soups, stews, and casseroles can be portioned and frozen for quick meals on busy days. Smoothie packs with pre-portioned fruits and vegetables can be assembled and frozen, ready to be blended with your choice of liquid for an instant nutritious breakfast or snack.

By thoughtfully stocking your fridge and freezer with these healthy essentials, you'll set yourself up for success in your healthy cooking journey. Remember to regularly rotate your items, using older products first and restocking as needed. With a well-stocked fridge and freezer, you'll always have the ingredients on hand to create nutritious, delicious meals, no matter how hectic your schedule may be.

Necessary Cooking Tools and Equipment

Having the right tools and equipment in your kitchen is just as important as stocking it with healthy ingredients. The proper utensils and appliances can make healthy cooking more efficient, enjoyable, and even more nutritious by allowing you to prepare foods in ways that preserve their nutrients. While it's not necessary to have every gadget on the market, investing in a few key pieces can significantly enhance your healthy cooking experience.

Let's start with the basics. A set of high-quality, sharp knives is essential for any kitchen. At minimum, you should have a chef's knife for general chopping and slicing, a paring knife for more delicate tasks, and a serrated knife for bread and tomatoes. Good knives make food preparation safer and more efficient, allowing you to chop vegetables and fruits with ease. Remember to keep your knives sharp, as dull knives can be dangerous and make food prep more difficult.

Cutting boards are another crucial item. It's advisable to have at least two: one for fruits and vegetables, and another for raw meats to prevent cross-contamination. Wooden or bamboo boards are gentle on knife edges and have natural antimicrobial properties, while plastic boards are dishwasher safe and easy to sanitize. Regardless of the material, make sure your cutting boards are sturdy and have non-slip features for safety.

When it comes to cookware, invest in a few versatile pieces that can handle a variety of cooking methods. A large, heavy-bottomed pot is perfect for soups, stews, and cooking grains. A non-stick skillet is useful for cooking eggs and delicate fish without adding excessive oil. Cast iron skillets are excellent for searing meats and vegetables, and they can go from stovetop to oven. Stainless steel pans are great for browning and creating flavorful sauces. Having a mix of these materials allows you to choose the best tool for each cooking task.

Bakeware is essential even if you're not a frequent baker. A couple of baking sheets are useful for roasting vegetables, a healthy cooking method that enhances flavor without adding extra fats. A *9*x*13* inch baking dish can be used for casseroles, baked fish dishes, and even roasting a whole chicken. Muffin tins are great for portion control, allowing you to make individual frittatas or baked oatmeal cups.

When it comes to small appliances, a food processor or high-powered blender can be a game-winner in a healthy kitchen. These versatile tools can be used to make smoothies, homemade nut butters, sauces, and even to chop vegetables quickly. They're particularly useful for creating creamy textures in dishes without relying on dairy products, which is beneficial for those following plant-based or dairy-free diets.

An immersion blender is another handy tool that takes up little space but offers big benefits. It's perfect for pureeing soups directly in the pot, making homemade salad dressings, or quickly blending a single-serve smoothie. This tool can help you create smooth, creamy textures without the need for cream or excessive fats.

A slow cooker or Instant Pot can be a valuable addition to your kitchen, especially if you have a busy lifestyle. These appliances allow you to prepare healthy, home-cooked meals with minimal hands-on time. They're great for cooking beans from scratch, making bone broth, or preparing large batches of soups and stews that can be portioned and frozen for future meals.

For those who enjoy homemade baked goods, a kitchen scale can be invaluable. Measuring ingredients by weight rather than volume is more accurate and can lead to better results, especially in baking. It's also helpful for portion control and can aid in tracking macronutrients if that's part of your health goals.

Don't overlook the importance of good measuring tools. A set of measuring cups and spoons for dry ingredients, and a glass measuring cup for liquids, will ensure accuracy in your cooking and baking. This is particularly important when you're adapting recipes to be healthier, as precise measurements can affect the outcome of the dish.

A salad spinner might seem like a luxury, but it's incredibly useful for washing and drying leafy greens and herbs. Properly dried greens stay fresh longer in the refrigerator and are more likely to be used in meals. Plus, salad dressings adhere better to dry leaves, meaning you can use less dressing while still getting great flavor.

Lastly, invest in a good set of storage containers. Glass containers with airtight lids are ideal for storing leftovers, prepped ingredients, and batch-cooked meals. They're safe for use in the microwave and don't absorb flavors or stains like plastic can. Having a variety of sizes allows you to store different portions efficiently, reducing food waste and making it easier to grab healthy meals and snacks throughout the week.

Remember, you don't need to acquire all these tools at once. Start with the basics and gradually add pieces as your cooking skills and needs evolve. The goal is to create a kitchen that supports and encourages your healthy cooking habits, making it easier and more enjoyable to prepare nutritious meals at home.

Healthy Ingredient Substitutions

One of the keys to successful healthy cooking is knowing how to make smart ingredient substitutions. By swapping out less nutritious ingredients for healthier alternatives, you can significantly improve the nutritional profile of your meals without sacrificing flavor or texture. These substitutions can help reduce calories, increase fiber and nutrient content, and make your favorite recipes more aligned with your health goals. Let's explore some versatile and effective healthy ingredient substitutions that you can incorporate into your cooking.

First, let's consider flour substitutions. While all-purpose white flour is a staple in many kitchens, it's often stripped of nutrients and fiber. Whole wheat flour is an excellent alternative that retains more of the grain's nutritional value. It can be used in most recipes that call for all-purpose flour, though you may need to adjust the liquid content slightly. For those avoiding gluten, almond flour or coconut flour can be good options, particularly in baking. These flours are higher in protein and healthy fats, and lower in carbohydrates compared to wheat flour. However, they behave differently in recipes, so it's best to follow recipes specifically designed for these flours or to experiment in small batches until you get the desired results.

When it comes to dairy, there are numerous healthy substitutions available. For milk, plant-based alternatives like almond milk, soy milk, or oat milk can be used in most recipes. These options are often lower in calories and saturated fat than whole milk, and many are fortified with calcium and vitamin *D*. In baking, unsweetened applesauce or mashed bananas can often replace some or all of the butter, reducing fat and adding natural sweetness and moisture. Greek yogurt is another versatile substitute that can replace sour cream in dips and dressings, or even butter in some baking recipes, adding protein and probiotics to your dishes.

Sugar is often overused in recipes, but there are many ways to reduce sugar content or use healthier alternatives. In baking, you can often reduce the sugar by *1/4* to *1/3* without significantly affecting the texture or taste. Natural sweeteners like mashed bananas, unsweetened applesauce, or dates can add sweetness while also contributing fiber and nutrients. Stevia, a natural zero-calorie sweetener, can be used in small amounts to add sweetness without calories. However, it's important to note that stevia is much sweeter than sugar, so you'll need to adjust the quantity accordingly.

For those looking to reduce meat consumption or follow a plant-based diet, there are numerous substitutions available. Lentils or mushrooms can replace some or all of the ground meat in recipes like burgers or meatloaf, adding fiber and reducing saturated fat. Tofu or tempeh can be marinated and used in place of chicken in many dishes. For eggs in baking, a "flax egg" (ground flaxseed mixed with water) can often be used as a binding agent, adding healthy omega-*3* fatty acids to your baked goods.

When it comes to fats and oils, there are several healthier options to consider. Avocado can be used as a spread in place of butter or mayonnaise, adding healthy monounsaturated fats and fiber. In baking, unsweetened applesauce or mashed bananas can often replace some or all of the oil, reducing fat content while maintaining moisture. When oil is necessary, choose healthier options like olive oil or avocado oil instead of vegetable or canola oil. These oils are rich in monounsaturated fats and have potential health benefits.

For those watching their carbohydrate intake, vegetable-based substitutions can be incredibly useful. Zucchini noodles or spaghetti squash can replace pasta in many dishes, significantly reducing calories and carbohydrates while increasing vegetable intake. Cauliflower rice is an excellent low-carb substitute for regular rice and can be used in stir-fries, burrito bowls, or as a side dish. Lettuce leaves can replace tortillas or bread in wraps and sandwiches, adding crunch and freshness while reducing calories.

In recipes that call for breading, consider using crushed nuts or seeds instead of breadcrumbs. This substitution adds healthy fats and protein while reducing refined carbohydrates. Almond meal or ground flaxseed can work well for this purpose. For a lower-calorie option, nutritional yeast can provide a savory, cheesy flavor without the added fat of cheese.

When it comes to condiments and sauces, there are many opportunities for healthy substitutions. Greek yogurt can replace mayonnaise in many dips and dressings, adding protein and probiotics. Mashed avocado can also serve as a creamy base for dressings. For a lower-calorie option, try using mustard or vinegar-based dressings instead of creamy ones. In recipes that call for cream, pureed white beans or cashew cream can often be used as a substitute, adding fiber and nutrients while reducing saturated fat.

Remember, when making substitutions, it's often best to start small and gradually increase the amount of the substitute used. This allows you to adjust to the new flavors and textures without dramatically altering your favorite recipes. Also, keep in mind that while these substitutions can make your meals healthier, they may slightly alter the taste or texture of the final dish. Embrace these changes as part of your journey towards healthier eating, and don't be afraid to experiment to find the substitutions that work best for you and your taste preferences.

By incorporating these healthy ingredient substitutions into your cooking, you can significantly improve the nutritional profile of your meals without feeling deprived. These swaps allow you to continue enjoying your favorite recipes while aligning them more closely with your health goals.

As you become more comfortable with these substitutions, you'll find that healthy cooking becomes second nature, opening up a world of delicious and nutritious possibilities in your kitchen.

Chapter 4: Mastering Healthy Cooking Techniques

Mastering healthy cooking techniques is essential for creating nutritious and delicious meals that support your well-being. By understanding and implementing these methods, you can enhance the flavor of your dishes while preserving their nutritional value. This chapter will explore five key cooking techniques that form the foundation of healthy cuisine: steaming, roasting, grilling, sautéing, and slow cooking. Each of these methods offers unique benefits and can be applied to a wide variety of ingredients, allowing you to create diverse and satisfying meals.

As you delve into these techniques, you'll discover how they can transform simple ingredients into extraordinary dishes. You'll learn how to retain vitamins and minerals, reduce the need for added fats, and bring out the natural flavors of foods. Moreover, you'll gain the confidence to experiment with different cooking methods, adapting them to suit your taste preferences and dietary needs. By the end of this chapter, you'll have a robust toolkit of cooking techniques at your disposal, enabling you to approach meal preparation with creativity and nutritional awareness.

Steaming: Preserving Nutrients and Flavor

Steaming is a gentle cooking method that uses hot water vapor to cook food, making it one of the healthiest ways to prepare meals. This technique is particularly effective for preserving the nutrients, color, and texture of vegetables, fish, and lean meats. When you steam food, it retains more vitamins and minerals compared to boiling or frying, as the nutrients are not leached into the cooking water or destroyed by high heat. Additionally, steaming requires no added fats, making it an excellent choice for those looking to reduce calorie intake without sacrificing flavor.

To start steaming, you'll need a steamer basket or a dedicated steaming appliance. If you don't have either, you can create a makeshift steamer by placing a heat-proof plate on top of a pot with a small amount of boiling water, ensuring the plate doesn't touch the water. Cover the pot with a tight-fitting lid to trap the steam. When steaming vegetables, it's crucial to avoid overcooking, as this can lead to nutrient loss and a mushy texture. As a general rule, most vegetables will steam to perfection in *5 -7* minutes, while denser vegetables like carrots or potatoes may require *10-15* minutes.

Steaming is particularly beneficial for leafy greens and cruciferous vegetables like broccoli and cauliflower. These vegetables retain more of their cancer-fighting compounds when steamed compared to other cooking methods[3]. For example, steamed broccoli retains up to *80%* of its glucosinolates, compounds associated with cancer prevention, compared to only *30%* when boiled.

To enhance the flavor of steamed foods without adding excess calories, consider using herbs, spices, or citrus zest. You can add these directly to the steaming water or sprinkle them over the food before steaming. For instance, adding lemon slices and dill to the steamer basket when cooking fish can infuse it with a delicate, aromatic flavor. Another technique is to use flavored liquids instead of plain water for steaming. Green tea, vegetable broth, or white wine can impart subtle flavors to your steamed dishes.

Steaming is not limited to vegetables and fish; it's also an excellent method for cooking whole grains and legumes. Quinoa, rice, and lentils can be steamed to fluffy perfection, often with better texture than when boiled. To steam grains, place them in a heat-proof bowl inside your steamer basket, add the appropriate amount of water or broth directly to the grains, and steam until tender. This method allows the grains to cook evenly without becoming waterlogged.

For those interested in Asian cuisine, steaming is a cornerstone technique. Dim sum, for example, showcases a variety of steamed dumplings and buns. You can create healthier versions of these dishes at home by using whole grain wrappers and lean protein fillings. Steamed bao buns filled with vegetables and lean meats offer a satisfying meal that's lower in calories and fat compared to their fried counterparts.

When it comes to meal planning, steaming can be a time-efficient cooking method. Many steamers come with multiple tiers, allowing you to cook several components of your meal simultaneously. For instance, you could steam fish on one level, vegetables on another, and grains on a third, creating a complete meal with minimal effort and equipment. This approach not only saves time but also reduces energy consumption in the kitchen.

To further maximize the nutritional benefits of steaming, consider consuming the cooking liquid. The small amount of water used in steaming often contains water-soluble vitamins and minerals that have leached out of the food. This nutrient-rich liquid can be used as a base for soups, sauces, or simply drunk as a nourishing broth. By utilizing this often-discarded liquid, you're ensuring that you're getting the full nutritional benefit of your steamed foods.

As you incorporate steaming into your cooking routine, remember that timing is crucial. Over-steaming can lead to loss of nutrients, flavor, and texture. It's better to slightly under-cook your food and then check for doneness, as you can always steam for an additional minute or two if needed. With practice, you'll develop an intuitive sense of steaming times for different foods, allowing you to consistently produce perfectly cooked, nutrient-rich meals.

Roasting: Enhancing Taste without Added Fats

Roasting is a dry-heat cooking method that can transform ingredients by caramelizing their natural sugars and concentrating their flavors, all while requiring minimal added fats. This technique is particularly effective for vegetables, lean meats, and even fruits, creating dishes with complex flavors and satisfying textures. Roasting typically involves cooking food in an oven at temperatures between 375°F and 425°F (190°C to 218°C), allowing the heat to envelop the food and cook it evenly.

One of the key benefits of roasting is its ability to enhance the natural sweetness of vegetables. When exposed to high heat, the sugars in vegetables caramelize, creating a depth of flavor that's difficult to achieve with other cooking methods. This makes roasting an excellent technique for making vegetables more appealing, especially for those who might not typically enjoy them. For instance, roasted Brussels sprouts develop a nutty, sweet flavor that's far removed from their often-maligned boiled counterpart.

To achieve the best results when roasting vegetables, it's important to cut them into uniform pieces to ensure even cooking. Toss the vegetables with a small amount of heart-healthy oil, such as olive or avocado oil, which helps to conduct heat and promote browning. Spread the vegetables in a single layer on a baking sheet, ensuring they're not overcrowded. Overcrowding can lead to steaming rather than roasting, resulting in less flavor development and a softer texture.

Roasting is also an excellent method for cooking lean meats and fish. Unlike frying, which often requires significant amounts of oil, roasting allows excess fat to drip away from the meat as it cooks. This results in a lower-fat final product without sacrificing flavor or moisture. When roasting meats, consider using a rack inside your roasting pan to elevate the meat and allow air to circulate, promoting even cooking and further fat reduction.

To enhance the nutritional value of roasted foods, consider incorporating herbs and spices. Not only do these add flavor without calories, but many herbs and spices also offer health benefits of their own. For example, rosemary, which pairs beautifully with roasted potatoes and chicken, contains compounds that may help improve digestion and boost the immune system[4]. Experiment with different herb and spice combinations to create diverse flavor profiles in your roasted dishes.

One often overlooked aspect of roasting is its potential for meal preparation. Roasting large batches of vegetables at the beginning of the week can provide you with versatile ingredients for multiple meals. These roasted vegetables can be used in salads, grain bowls, sandwiches, or as side dishes, saving time and ensuring you always have a nutritious option on hand. Similarly, roasting a whole chicken can provide lean protein for several meals, from sandwiches to salads to soups.

When it comes to roasting fruits, this technique can create unique dessert options that are lower in added sugars compared to traditional sweets. Roasting intensifies the natural sweetness of fruits like peaches, pears, and plums, creating a caramelized exterior and a soft, juicy interior. These roasted fruits can be served on their own, paired with a small scoop of yogurt, or used as a topping for oatmeal or whole grain pancakes.

To maximize the nutritional benefits of roasting, it's important to be mindful of cooking temperatures and times. While high heat is necessary for browning and flavor development, excessive heat or prolonged cooking can lead to the formation of potentially harmful compounds, particularly in meat. To mitigate this, consider marinating meats before roasting, as the antioxidants in marinades can help reduce the formation of these compounds[5].

Roasting can also be an energy-efficient cooking method, especially when preparing multiple components of a meal simultaneously. By utilizing the entire oven space and cooking several items at once, you can reduce overall energy consumption and cooking time. For instance, you might roast a tray of vegetables on one rack, a piece of fish on another, and even include a tray of fruit for dessert, all cooking at the same temperature.

As you incorporate roasting into your healthy cooking repertoire, remember that it's a versatile technique that can be adapted to suit various dietary needs. For those following a plant-based diet, roasted vegetables can form the centerpiece of a meal, offering satisfying textures and flavors that can rival meat-based dishes. For those monitoring their carbohydrate intake, roasting low-carb vegetables like cauliflower, zucchini, or bell peppers can create satisfying side dishes or even main course options.

Grilling: Healthy Outdoor Cooking

Grilling is a cooking method that not only imparts a unique, smoky flavor to food but also offers several health benefits when done correctly. This technique involves cooking food over direct heat, typically on a barbecue grill or a grill pan. Grilling is particularly effective for reducing the fat content of meats, as excess fat drips away from the food during cooking. Additionally, the high heat used in grilling can help seal in moisture and flavors, reducing the need for added fats or sauces.

One of the primary advantages of grilling is its ability to enhance the natural flavors of foods without relying on excessive oils or butter. The intense heat caramelizes the surface of meats, vegetables, and even fruits, creating complex flavor profiles and appealing textures. For example, grilled pineapple develops a sweet-smoky taste that can serve as a healthier dessert option or a unique addition to savory dishes.

When grilling meats, it's important to choose lean cuts to maximize the health benefits. Skinless chicken breast, fish, and lean cuts of beef or pork are excellent options. Marinating these meats before grilling can not only enhance flavor but also provide health benefits. Studies have shown that marinating meat in mixtures containing herbs and spices can reduce the formation of potentially harmful compounds during high-heat cooking[6].

Grilling vegetables is an excellent way to increase their appeal and consumption. The high heat of grilling caramelizes the natural sugars in vegetables, creating a sweet and smoky flavor that can make even the most vegetable-averse individuals reconsider their stance. Vegetables like zucchini, eggplant, bell peppers, and asparagus are particularly well-suited to grilling. To prevent sticking and ensure even cooking, lightly brush vegetables with a small amount of olive oil before placing them on the grill.

For those following a plant-based diet, grilling can offer exciting possibilities. Firm tofu, tempeh, and seitan can be marinated and grilled to create satisfying meat alternatives. Grilled portobello mushrooms, with their meaty texture and ability to absorb flavors, can serve as an excellent substitute for burger patties. These options not only provide protein but also offer a range of nutrients and fiber not found in animal-based products.

When it comes to grilling fish, this method can help retain more omega-*3* fatty acids compared to frying. Omega-*3*s are essential for heart and brain health, and grilling helps preserve these beneficial compounds. Delicate fish like salmon or trout can be grilled on cedar planks, which not only prevents the fish from sticking to the grill but also imparts a subtle woody flavor to the dish.

To further enhance the nutritional value of grilled foods, consider incorporating a variety of herbs and spices into your marinades or rubs. These not only add flavor without calories but also provide additional health benefits. For instance, rosemary and thyme contain antioxidants that can help counteract some of the potentially harmful effects of high-heat cooking[7].

Grilling can also be an excellent method for preparing fruit-based desserts. Grilled peaches, nectarines, or pineapple slices can be served with a small dollop of Greek yogurt and a drizzle of honey for a healthier dessert option. The grilling process caramelizes the natural sugars in the fruit, intensifying their sweetness without the need for added sugars.

While grilling offers many health benefits, it's important to be mindful of certain precautions. High-heat cooking methods like grilling can lead to the formation of potentially harmful compounds, particularly when meat is charred. To minimize this risk, avoid charring your food and consider using a marinade, which can reduce the formation of these compounds by up to *88%*[8]. Additionally, flipping meat frequently during grilling can help reduce the formation of these compounds.

Grilling can also be a social and enjoyable way to prepare meals, encouraging outdoor dining and physical activity. This social aspect of grilling can contribute to overall well-being, as sharing meals with others has been linked to improved mental health and better eating habits. Consider organizing healthy grill-outs with friends and family, featuring a variety of grilled vegetables, lean proteins, and fruit-based desserts.

As you incorporate grilling into your healthy cooking routine, remember that it's a versatile technique that can be adapted to various dietary needs and preferences. Whether you're grilling vegetables for a vegan feast, preparing lean meats for a high-protein meal, or creating fruit-based desserts for a low-sugar option, grilling offers endless possibilities for creating delicious and nutritious dishes.

Sautéing: Quick and Flavorful Cooking

Sautéing is a versatile and efficient cooking technique that involves cooking food quickly in a small amount of oil over relatively high heat. This method is particularly useful for busy individuals looking to prepare healthy meals without spending hours in the kitchen. Sautéing allows you to cook foods rapidly while preserving their nutrients, texture, and flavor, making it an excellent choice for both vegetables and lean proteins.

One of the key advantages of sautéing is its ability to cook food quickly while retaining nutritional value. The short cooking time and minimal use of liquid help preserve water-soluble vitamins that might otherwise be lost during longer cooking processes or methods that involve submerging food in water. For example, sautéed spinach retains more of its folate content compared to boiled spinach[9].

To sauté effectively, start by choosing the right pan. A wide, shallow pan with sloped sides, such as a sauté pan or a large skillet, is ideal. This design allows for easy tossing and stirring of ingredients. The pan should be large enough to accommodate your ingredients in a single layer, as overcrowding can lead to steaming rather than sautéing, resulting in less flavor development and potentially soggy textures.

When it comes to oil selection for sautéing, opt for oils with high smoke points and beneficial nutritional profiles. Extra virgin olive oil, avocado oil, and grapeseed oil are excellent choices. These oils can withstand the high heat of sautéing without breaking down and producing harmful compounds. Moreover, they offer heart-healthy monounsaturated fats. Use oil sparingly; typically, one to two tablespoons is sufficient for a four-serving recipe.

Sautéing is particularly effective for cooking vegetables. The high heat and quick cooking time help vegetables retain their crisp texture and vibrant colors. Start by sautéing aromatics like garlic and onions to build a flavor base, then add harder vegetables like carrots or bell peppers, followed by more delicate vegetables like leafy greens. This layered approach ensures that each ingredient is cooked to perfection.

For those looking to increase their vegetable intake, sautéing can make vegetables more appealing by enhancing their natural flavors and creating interesting textures. Consider experimenting with less common vegetables like bok choy, fennel, or kohlrabi. Sautéing these vegetables can introduce new flavors and textures to your meals, helping to diversify your nutrient intake.

When sautéing proteins, such as chicken breast or tofu, it's important to ensure the pan is hot before adding the food. This helps create a flavorful crust on the exterior while keeping the interior moist. For even cooking, cut proteins into uniform pieces. Consider dusting lean meats or tofu with a small amount of whole wheat flour or cornstarch before sautéing; this can help create a crispy exterior without the need for excessive oil.

To further enhance the nutritional value of sautéed dishes, incorporate herbs and spices. Not only do these add flavor without calories, but many also offer health benefits. For instance, turmeric, which pairs well with sautéed vegetables and lean proteins, contains curcumin, a compound with potent anti-inflammatory properties[10]. Adding fresh herbs towards the end of cooking can provide a burst of flavor and additional nutrients.

Sautéing can also be an excellent method for preparing quick, healthy stir-fries. These dishes typically combine a variety of vegetables with a lean protein source, creating a balanced meal in a single pan. To keep stir-fries healthy, use minimal oil and focus on loading the dish with a variety of colorful vegetables. For the sauce, opt for low-sodium soy sauce or create your own using ingredients like rice vinegar, ginger, and a small amount of honey for sweetness.

For those following specific dietary patterns, sautéing can be easily adapted. Plant-based eaters can sauté tofu, tempeh, or seitan as protein sources, while those following low-carb diets can focus on sautéing non-starchy vegetables and lean proteins. The versatility of this cooking method allows for endless combinations and adaptations to suit various nutritional needs and preferences.

While sautéing is generally a healthy cooking method, it's important to be mindful of the amount of oil used. Even healthy oils are calorie-dense, so using them judiciously is key to maintaining a balanced diet. One technique to reduce oil usage is to use a non-stick pan or a well-seasoned cast-iron skillet, which require less oil to prevent sticking.

Incorporating sautéing into your meal prep routine can significantly streamline your cooking process. Consider sautéing a large batch of mixed vegetables at the beginning of the week. These can be stored in the refrigerator and quickly reheated for use in salads, grain bowls, or as side dishes throughout the week. This approach not only saves time but also ensures you always have a healthy vegetable option ready to go.

As you become more comfortable with sautéing, you can start experimenting with more complex flavor profiles. Try combining different cuisines by using spice blends from various culinary traditions. For example, you might sauté vegetables with Moroccan spices one day and Indian curry blends the next, creating diverse and exciting meals using the same basic technique.

Slow Cooking: Convenience and Nutrition

Slow cooking is a method that combines convenience with nutrition, allowing you to create flavorful, nutrient-rich meals with minimal effort. This technique involves cooking food at low temperatures for extended periods, typically using a slow cooker or crockpot. Slow cooking is particularly beneficial for busy individuals who want to ensure they have healthy, home-cooked meals despite time constraints. It's also an excellent way to make tougher, less expensive cuts of meat tender and delicious, while retaining and even enhancing their nutritional value.

One of the primary advantages of slow cooking is its ability to preserve nutrients in food. The low, steady heat and moisture-rich environment of a slow cooker help retain water-soluble vitamins and minerals that might be lost in other high-heat cooking methods. For example, slow-cooked vegetables often retain more of their vitamin *C* content compared to boiled or steamed vegetables[11].

Slow cooking is particularly effective for preparing lean meats and tough cuts. The long, slow cooking process breaks down connective tissues in meat, resulting in tender, flavorful dishes without the need for added fats. This makes it an excellent method for cooking lean cuts of beef, pork, or chicken, as well as plant-based protein sources like beans and lentils. The moist cooking environment also helps prevent the formation of potentially harmful compounds that can occur with high-heat cooking methods.

When using a slow cooker, it's important to layer ingredients properly to ensure even cooking. Start by placing harder vegetables like carrots, potatoes, and onions at the bottom of the pot, as they take longer to cook. Add meat next, followed by more delicate vegetables and any liquids. This layering technique allows flavors to meld while ensuring each ingredient is cooked to the right consistency.

Slow cooking is an excellent way to incorporate more vegetables into your diet. The long cooking time allows vegetables to become tender and absorb the flavors of the dish, making them more appealing even to those who might not typically enjoy them. Consider adding a variety of colorful vegetables to your slow cooker meals to increase your nutrient intake and add texture to your dishes.

For those following specific dietary patterns, slow cooking can be easily adapted. Plant-based eaters can use slow cookers to prepare hearty vegetable stews, bean dishes, or meat alternatives like jackfruit. Those on low-carb diets can focus on meat and low-carb vegetable combinations. The versatility of slow cooking allows for endless combinations to suit various nutritional needs and preferences.

Slow cooking can also be an excellent method for preparing large batches of food for meal prepping. A single slow cooker meal can often provide several servings, which can be portioned out for lunches or dinners throughout the week. This not only saves time but also ensures you have healthy, home-cooked meals readily available, reducing the temptation to opt for less nutritious convenience foods.

When it comes to flavoring slow cooker meals, herbs and spices play a crucial role. Unlike stovetop cooking where flavors can evaporate, the sealed environment of a slow cooker allows spices to infuse deeply into the food. This means you can use less salt while still creating flavorful dishes. Consider using herbs like rosemary, thyme, and bay leaves, which stand up well to long cooking times and impart robust flavors.

Slow cooking is particularly beneficial for preparing nutrient-dense bone broths and stocks. These liquids, rich in minerals and collagen, can be used as bases for soups and stews or consumed on their own for their potential health benefits. The long, slow simmering process extracts maximum nutrients from bones and vegetables, creating a nourishing liquid that's easy to digest and full of flavor.

For those concerned about the safety of leaving appliances on for extended periods, modern slow cookers are designed with safety features that make them suitable for all-day cooking. However, it's important to follow food safety guidelines, such as avoiding the addition of frozen ingredients and ensuring meats reach safe internal temperatures.

While slow cooking is generally a healthy method, it's important to be mindful of the ingredients used. Avoid adding excessive amounts of high-fat or high-sodium ingredients. Instead, focus on lean proteins, plenty of vegetables, and moderate amounts of whole grains. If a recipe calls for cream or cheese, consider using low-fat alternatives or reducing the amount used.

Slow cooking can also be an energy-efficient cooking method, especially when compared to using an oven for extended periods. This can be particularly beneficial during hot summer months when you want to avoid heating up your kitchen. Additionally, the ability to cook large batches at once can reduce overall energy consumption compared to cooking multiple smaller meals.

As you incorporate slow cooking into your healthy cooking routine, remember that it's a method that rewards experimentation. Don't be afraid to adapt recipes to suit your tastes and nutritional needs. You might find that certain ingredients you typically don't enjoy becoming more palatable when slow-cooked, opening up new possibilities for variety in your diet. With practice, you'll develop an intuitive understanding of how different ingredients behave in a slow cooker, allowing you to create your own nutritious and delicious recipes.

Chapter 5: Effective Meal Planning and Prep

Effective meal planning and preparation are the cornerstones of maintaining a healthy diet and lifestyle. By taking the time to plan your meals and prepare ingredients in advance (which I don't recommend unless you need to), you can ensure that you're consistently eating nutritious, balanced meals throughout the week. This chapter will guide you through the process of creating a weekly meal plan, developing efficient grocery shopping strategies, mastering batch cooking techniques, and implementing proper food storage practices. These skills will not only save you time and reduce stress but also help you make healthier food choices and minimize food waste.

Creating a Weekly Meal Plan

A well-structured weekly meal plan is the foundation of successful healthy eating. It helps you stay organized, saves time, reduces stress, and ensures that you have a balanced diet throughout the week. To create an effective meal plan, start by setting aside some time each week, preferably on a weekend or a day when you have fewer commitments. This dedicated planning session will allow you to thoughtfully consider your nutritional needs, preferences, and schedule for the upcoming week.

Begin by assessing your calendar for the week ahead. Take note of any special events, late work nights, or other commitments that might affect your mealtimes or cooking availability. This awareness will help you plan realistically and avoid the temptation to resort to unhealthy convenience foods when time is tight. Next, consider your nutritional goals and dietary preferences. Are you aiming to increase your vegetable intake? Trying to incorporate more lean proteins? Or perhaps you're looking to experiment with new whole grains? Keep these objectives in mind as you plan your meals.

When selecting recipes for your meal plan, aim for a balance of familiar favorites and new dishes to keep things interesting. Consider recipes that share common ingredients to minimize waste and streamline your grocery shopping. For example, if you're planning to make a stir-fry with bell peppers one night, you might incorporate the leftover peppers into a salad or omelet later in the week. Also, think about how you can repurpose leftovers creatively. A grilled chicken breast from Monday's dinner could become part of Tuesday's lunch salad or Wednesday's wrap.

As you plan, don't forget to include all meals and snacks. While dinner often gets the most attention, planning for breakfast, lunch, and healthy snacks is equally important for maintaining a balanced diet. Consider prepping some grab-and-go breakfast options like overnight oats or egg muffins for busy mornings. For lunches, think about meals that can be easily packed and transported if you're eating away from home.

Once you've outlined your meals for the week, create a comprehensive grocery list based on your plan. Organize your list by store sections (produce, dairy, grains, etc.) to make your shopping trip more efficient. This approach not only saves time at the store but also helps you avoid impulse purchases that might not align with your healthy eating goals.

Remember that flexibility is key when it comes to meal planning. While having a structured plan is beneficial, it's important to allow for some adaptability. You might want to leave one or two meals open for using up leftovers or accommodating unexpected changes in your schedule. The goal is to create a plan that supports your healthy eating goals while still being realistic and enjoyable.

To make the meal planning process even more efficient, consider using digital tools or apps designed for this purpose. Many of these tools allow you to save favorite recipes, generate grocery lists automatically, and even plan meals based on sales at your local grocery stores. Experiment with different methods and find a system that works best for you. Some people prefer a physical planner or whiteboard, while others might opt for a digital solution.

As you become more comfortable with meal planning, you'll likely start to notice patterns in your eating habits and preferences. Use this information to streamline your planning process further. For example, you might find that having a theme for each day of the week (like Meatless Monday or Stir-Fry Friday) helps simplify decision-making. Or you might discover that batch cooking certain staples on the weekend sets you up for easier meal assembly during the week.

Lastly, don't forget to involve your family or household members in the meal planning process if applicable. Getting input from others can help ensure that everyone's preferences and nutritional needs are considered, increasing the likelihood that the meals will be enjoyed and reducing food waste. It can also be an opportunity to educate children about nutrition and involve them in making healthy food choices.

By consistently practicing and refining your meal planning skills, you'll find that it becomes an integral part of your healthy lifestyle. A well-thought-out meal plan not only supports your nutritional goals but also reduces the stress and decision fatigue often associated with daily meal choices. With time, you'll develop a repertoire of go-to meals and a streamlined planning process that makes healthy eating a natural and enjoyable part of your routine.

Efficient Grocery Shopping Strategies

Efficient grocery shopping is a crucial skill that complements your meal planning efforts and supports your healthy eating goals. By developing smart shopping strategies, you can save time, money, and ensure that your kitchen is stocked with nutritious ingredients. The key to efficient grocery shopping lies in preparation, organization, and mindful decision-making while in the store.

Start by creating a detailed grocery list based on your meal plan. Organize this list by store sections (produce, dairy, grains, etc.) to streamline your shopping experience. This approach not only saves time but also helps you avoid wandering through aisles unnecessarily, which can lead to impulse purchases. Consider using a grocery list app on your smartphone, which can allow you to easily add items throughout the week as you notice you're running low. Some apps even allow you to share lists with family members, ensuring that everyone can contribute to the household shopping needs.

Before heading to the store, take inventory of what you already have in your pantry, refrigerator, and freezer. This step prevents you from buying duplicates and helps you plan meals that use up ingredients you already have on hand, reducing food waste. It's also a good idea to check for any coupons or store promotions that align with your shopping list. However, be cautious about buying items solely because they're on sale – stick to your list and your nutritional goals.

When you arrive at the store, start with the perimeter last. This is where you'll typically find fresh produce, lean meats, dairy, and other whole foods. These unprocessed or minimally processed foods should form the foundation of your healthy diet. As you select produce, choose a variety of colorful fruits and vegetables to ensure a wide range of nutrients. Don't shy away from frozen fruits and vegetables, which can be just as nutritious as fresh and often more convenient and cost-effective.

As you're in the store, read nutrition labels carefully. Pay attention to serving sizes, calorie content, and the amounts of added sugars, sodium, and unhealthy fats. Look for products with shorter ingredient lists, focusing on whole food ingredients you recognize. Be wary of health claims on packaging – these can sometimes be misleading. Instead, rely on your knowledge of nutrition basics to make informed choices.

When shopping for grains, opt for whole grain versions of bread, pasta, and rice whenever possible. These provide more fiber and nutrients than their refined counterparts. In the protein section, choose lean meats, fish, and plant-based protein sources like beans and lentils. If you're buying canned goods, look for low-sodium options and those packed in water rather than oil or syrup.

Be strategic about when you shop. Try to avoid going to the grocery store when you're hungry, as this can lead to impulse purchases and unhealthy choices. If possible, shop during off-peak hours to avoid crowds and reduce stress. Some people find it helpful to do a larger shopping trip once a week, supplemented by quick trips for fresh produce mid-week.

Consider buying in bulk for non-perishable items and foods you use frequently. This can be more cost-effective and reduce packaging waste. However, be cautious about buying perishables in large quantities unless you're certain you'll use them before they spoil. For items with a longer shelf life, like grains or frozen vegetables, buying in bulk can be a great way to save money and ensure you always have healthy staples on hand.

Don't be afraid to try store brands or generic products, especially for staple items. These are often significantly cheaper than name brands and can be just as nutritious. Compare unit prices (price per ounce or per pound) rather than just the sticker price to ensure you're getting the best value.

As you become more familiar with your local grocery store's layout and offerings, you'll likely develop a routine that makes shopping even more efficient. You might find that certain days of the week have better produce selections or that specific stores are better for certain types of items. Use this knowledge to optimize your shopping strategy.

Remember that efficient grocery shopping is a skill that improves with practice. Over time, you'll become more adept at quickly selecting the best ingredients for your needs and budget. You'll also develop a better sense of how much food you need to buy to support your meal plan without overbuying and risking waste.

By implementing these efficient grocery shopping strategies, you'll not only save time and money but also set yourself up for success in your healthy cooking endeavors. A well-stocked kitchen with nutritious ingredients makes it much easier to stick to your meal plan and resist the temptation of less healthy convenience foods. With practice, grocery shopping can become an enjoyable part of your healthy lifestyle routine, rather than a chore.

Batch Cooking for Time Efficiency

Batch cooking (which I don't recommend unless you need to) can be a powerful strategy for maintaining your diet while managing a busy lifestyle. This technique involves preparing larger quantities of food at once, which can then be portioned out and used for multiple meals throughout the week. By dedicating a few hours to batch cooking, you can save significant time and energy on busy weekdays, making it easier to stick to your healthy eating goals.

To get started with batch cooking, choose a day when you have a few hours to spare, such as a weekend afternoon. Begin by selecting recipes that lend themselves well to batch cooking. Soups, stews, casseroles, and grain-based dishes are excellent options as they often taste even better after a day or two as flavors meld. Roasted vegetables, grilled chicken breasts, and cooked whole grains are also great candidates for batch preparation, as they can be easily incorporated into various meals throughout the week.

When planning your batch cooking session, consider how you can maximize efficiency in the kitchen. For example, while a pot of soup is simmering on the stove, you could be roasting vegetables in the oven and cooking a large batch of quinoa on another burner. This multitasking approach allows you to prepare several components of future meals simultaneously, significantly reducing overall cooking time.

As you cook, think about how the foods you're preparing can be used in different ways throughout the week. A large batch of roasted vegetables, for instance, could be used as a side dish one night, incorporated into a grain bowl for lunch the next day, and blended into a soup later in the week. This versatility not only saves time but also adds variety to your meals, preventing boredom with your healthy eating plan.

Proper storage is crucial for successful batch cooking. Invest in a set of high-quality, airtight containers in various sizes. Glass containers are ideal as they're microwave-safe and don't absorb flavors or odors. Portion out your prepared foods into meal-sized servings before storing. This step makes it easy to grab a single portion for lunch or quickly assemble dinner on busy evenings. Label each container with the contents and date prepared to keep track of freshness.

When it comes to storing batch-cooked meals, your freezer can be a valuable ally. Many dishes freeze well and can be safely stored for several months. Soups, stews, cooked grains, and casseroles are particularly freezer-friendly. To freeze effectively, allow foods to cool completely before packaging them in freezer-safe containers or bags. Remove as much air as possible to prevent freezer burn. Remember to label each item with the contents and date frozen.

While batch cooking can save significant time during the week, it's important to consider food safety. Cooked foods should be cooled quickly and stored in the refrigerator within two hours of cooking. Large batches of hot food should be divided into smaller portions to cool more rapidly. In the refrigerator, most cooked foods will stay fresh for *3-4* days. Beyond that, consider freezing for longer storage.

As you incorporate batch cooking into your routine, you'll likely discover which recipes and methods work best for you. Some people prefer to prepare complete meals in advance, while others find it more flexible to batch cook individual components (like grains, proteins, and vegetables) that can be mixed and matched throughout the week. Experiment with different approaches to find what suits your lifestyle and preferences.

Remember that batch cooking doesn't mean you have to eat the same thing every day. Use your prepared components creatively to assemble varied meals. For example, cooked chicken breast could be used in a salad one day, in a wrap the next, and in a stir-fry later in the week. This approach provides variety while still capitalizing on the time-saving benefits of batch cooking.

Batch cooking can also be a great opportunity to involve family members or roommates in meal preparation. Turn it into a social activity where everyone contributes to the cooking process. This not only makes the task more enjoyable but also ensures that the meals prepared will appeal to everyone's tastes.

By mastering the art of batch cooking, you're setting yourself up for success in your healthy eating journey. This time-efficient approach not only makes it easier to stick to your nutritional goals but also reduces the stress associated with daily meal preparation. With practice, you'll find that batch cooking becomes an integral part of your healthy lifestyle, allowing you to enjoy nutritious, home-cooked meals even on your busiest days.

Proper Food Storage Tips

Proper food storage is a crucial aspect of maintaining a healthy kitchen and maximizing the nutritional value of your ingredients. Effective storage not only extends the life of your food but also helps prevent foodborne illnesses and reduces waste. By mastering proper storage techniques, you can ensure that the nutritious ingredients you've carefully selected remain fresh and safe to eat for as long as possible.

Let's start with the refrigerator, which is the primary storage area for many perishable foods. The key to effective refrigerator storage is temperature control and organization. Your refrigerator should be set to 40°F (4°C) or below to slow bacterial growth and keep food fresh. Use a refrigerator thermometer to ensure your appliance is maintaining the correct temperature. Organize your refrigerator so that raw meats are stored on the bottom shelf to prevent any drips from contaminating other foods. Keep fruits and vegetables in the crisper drawers, where humidity levels can be controlled to extend their freshness.

Different types of produce have different storage needs. Some fruits, like apples and pears, release ethylene gas as they ripen, which can cause nearby produce to spoil more quickly. Store these fruits separately from ethylene-sensitive items like leafy greens. Many vegetables, such as carrots, celery, and broccoli, stay crisp longer when stored in water. Cut them into sticks and store in containers filled with water, changing the water every few days. Herbs can be treated like flowers - trim the stems and place them in a jar with water, then cover loosely with a plastic bag.

For dry goods and pantry items, the key factors are temperature, humidity, and protection from pests. Store these items in a cool, dry place away from direct sunlight. Airtight containers are essential for keeping out moisture and insects. Transfer items like flour, sugar, and grains to airtight containers as soon as you bring them home. This not only protects them from pests but also makes it easier to see when you're running low. Label containers with the contents and date of purchase to keep track of freshness.

The freezer is an excellent tool for long-term storage of many foods. Most foods can be frozen, but it's important to package them properly to prevent freezer burn. Remove as much air as possible from packaging before freezing. For liquids like soups or sauces, leave some headspace in the container as liquids expand when frozen. Label all frozen items with the contents and date frozen. As a general rule, most frozen foods remain safe indefinitely, but quality begins to decline after a few months.

When it comes to leftovers, proper storage is crucial for both safety and quality. Cool leftovers quickly by dividing large amounts into smaller, shallow containers. This allows the food to reach a safe temperature more rapidly. Once cooled, store leftovers in airtight containers in the refrigerator and use within *3-4* days. For longer storage, freeze leftovers in portion-sized containers for easy reheating.

Proper storage of oils and fats is often overlooked but important for maintaining their quality and preventing rancidity. Store cooking oils in a cool, dark place. Some oils, like olive oil, can be kept at room temperature, while others, particularly nut and seed oils, benefit from refrigeration. Butter can be kept at room temperature for a few days if you use it quickly, but for longer storage, keep it in the refrigerator or freezer.

For bread and baked goods, the storage method depends on how quickly you plan to use them. For short-term storage (within a few days), keep bread in a bread box or paper bag at room temperature. For longer storage, freeze bread in an airtight bag. Avoid storing bread in the refrigerator, as this can actually accelerate staling.

When storing fresh herbs, treat soft herbs (like basil, cilantro, and parsley) differently from hard herbs (like rosemary, thyme, and oregano). Soft herbs can be stored like flowers in a glass of water, covered loosely with a plastic bag, in the refrigerator. Hard herbs can be wrapped in slightly damp paper towels and stored in a plastic bag in the refrigerator.

For cheese, the key is to allow it to breathe while protecting it from drying out. Wrap cheese in wax paper or cheese paper, then loosely in plastic wrap. This allows excess moisture to escape while preventing the cheese from drying out completely. Store wrapped cheese in the vegetable crisper of your refrigerator, where the humidity is higher.

Remember that proper food storage begins at the grocery store. When shopping, pick up refrigerated and frozen items last to minimize the time they spend at room temperature. Use insulated bags for transporting these items home, especially in hot weather. Once home, put away perishable items first before dealing with pantry staples.

By implementing these proper food storage techniques, you'll not only extend the life of your ingredients but also ensure that they retain their nutritional value and flavor. This approach reduces food waste, saves money, and supports your efforts to maintain a healthy, well-stocked kitchen. With practice, proper food storage will become second nature, allowing you to effortlessly maintain a fresh and nutritious food supply for all your healthy cooking needs.

Chapter 6: Energizing Breakfast Recipes

Breakfast is often hailed as the most important meal of the day, and for good reason. A nutritious breakfast sets the tone for your entire day, providing the energy and nutrients your body needs to function optimally. In this chapter, we'll explore a variety of energizing breakfast recipes that not only taste delicious but also offer a balanced mix of nutrients to fuel your morning activities. From vibrant smoothie bowls to hearty savory options, these recipes are designed to kickstart your day with a boost of nutrition and flavor.

The importance of a healthy breakfast cannot be overstated. Research has consistently shown that people who eat a nutritious breakfast tend to have better overall diet quality, improved concentration and memory, and are more likely to maintain a healthy weight[12]. By incorporating a balance of complex carbohydrates, lean proteins, and healthy fats into your morning meal, you can stabilize blood sugar levels, reduce cravings throughout the day, and provide your body with sustained energy.

In this chapter, we'll delve into four key areas of breakfast preparation: nutrient-packed smoothie bowls, versatile overnight oats, savory breakfast options, and some quick and healthy breakfast ideas. Each section will provide you with a range of recipes and techniques to diversify your breakfast routine and ensure that you're starting your day on the right nutritional foot. Whether you're a busy professional looking for grab-and-go options or someone who enjoys a leisurely morning meal, you'll find recipes and ideas to suit your lifestyle and taste preferences.

As we explore these breakfast options, keep in mind that the recipes provided are flexible and can be adapted to suit your individual nutritional needs and preferences. Feel free to experiment with different ingredients, adjust portion sizes, or modify recipes to accommodate dietary restrictions. The goal is to create breakfast habits that are not only healthy but also enjoyable and sustainable for your lifestyle.

Nutrient-Packed Smoothie Bowls

Smoothie bowls have gained popularity in recent years, and for good reason. These vibrant, nutrient-dense creations offer a perfect balance of flavors, textures, and essential nutrients to start your day. Unlike traditional smoothies, smoothie bowls are thicker in consistency and are eaten with a spoon, allowing for the addition of crunchy toppings that add extra nutrition and satisfaction to your meal.

The base of a smoothie bowl typically consists of blended frozen fruits, which provide natural sweetness and a creamy texture without the need for added sugars. This frozen fruit base is often combined with a liquid such as plant-based milk, coconut water, or green tea, and can be fortified with nutrient-rich add-ins like leafy greens, chia seeds, or protein powder. The result is a thick, spoonable consistency that serves as the perfect canvas for an array of toppings.

One of the key benefits of smoothie bowls is their versatility. You can easily customize your bowl to meet specific nutritional goals or dietary preferences. For example, if you're looking to increase your protein intake, you might add a scoop of plant-based protein powder or Greek yogurt to your base. If you're aiming to boost your omega-*3* fatty acid intake, consider adding ground flaxseeds or chia seeds. The possibilities are virtually endless, allowing you to create a different nutritional profile each day based on your body's needs.

When creating your smoothie bowl, aim for a balance of macronutrients. Include a source of complex carbohydrates (such as fruits or oats), healthy fats (like nuts, seeds, or avocado), and protein (from Greek yogurt, protein powder, or nut butter). This balance will help keep you feeling full and energized throughout the morning. Additionally, the inclusion of fruits and vegetables in your smoothie bowl base provides essential vitamins, minerals, and fiber, contributing to your daily nutrient intake.

Here's a basic formula for creating a nutrient-packed smoothie bowl:

- Base: *1-2* cups frozen fruit (e.g., berries, banana, mango)
- Liquid: *1/2-1* cup liquid (e.g., almond milk, coconut water)

- Nutrient Boost: *1-2* tablespoons (e.g., chia seeds, protein powder, spinach)
- Toppings: *2-3* tablespoons of various toppings (e.g., granola, sliced fruit, nuts)

Let's explore a few nutrient-packed smoothie bowl recipes to get you started:

1. Berry Bliss Bowl:

- Base: *1* cup frozen mixed berries, *1/2* frozen banana
- Liquid: *1/2* cup unsweetened almond milk
- Nutrient Boost: *1* tablespoon chia seeds, *1* handful spinach
- Toppings: Sliced almonds, fresh berries, hemp seeds

2. Tropical Green Goddess Bowl:

- Base: *1* cup frozen mango, *1/2* frozen banana
- Liquid: *1/2* cup coconut water
- Nutrient Boost: *1* handful kale, *1* scoop vanilla protein powder
- Toppings: Coconut flakes, sliced kiwi, pumpkin seeds

3. Chocolate Peanut Butter Power Bowl:

- Base: 1 frozen banana, *1/2* cup frozen cauliflower rice (for added nutrients)
- Liquid: *3/4* cup unsweetened almond milk
- Nutrient Boost: *1* tablespoon unsweetened cocoa powder, *1* tablespoon peanut butter
- Toppings: Cacao nibs, sliced banana, chopped peanuts

When preparing your smoothie bowl, start by blending the frozen fruits with a small amount of liquid. Add more liquid gradually until you achieve a thick, spoonable consistency. It's important to use frozen fruits as they create a creamier texture and help keep the bowl cold, allowing you to take your time enjoying your breakfast. If your blender is struggling, stop and scrape down the sides, or add a little more liquid.

Remember, the key to a great smoothie bowl is not just in the base, but also in the toppings. Choose toppings that not only add nutritional value but also provide a variety of textures. Crunchy elements like granola or nuts can make your smoothie bowl more satisfying and enjoyable to eat. Fresh fruits can add a burst of flavor and additional nutrients, while seeds or nut butters can increase the protein and healthy fat content of your bowl.

By incorporating smoothie bowls into your breakfast routine, you're not only treating yourself to a delicious and visually appealing meal but also providing your body with a concentrated dose of nutrients to start your day. Experiment with different combinations of fruits, vegetables, and toppings to find your favorite variations, and don't be afraid to get creative with your presentations. A beautiful, nutrient-packed smoothie bowl can be a wonderful way to practice mindful eating and set a positive tone for the day ahead.

Versatile Overnight Oats

Overnight oats have become a breakfast staple for many health-conscious individuals, and for good reason. This simple, no-cook method of preparing oatmeal is not only convenient but also incredibly versatile, allowing for endless flavor combinations and nutritional customization. At its core, overnight oats are simply raw oats soaked in liquid overnight, resulting in a creamy, pudding-like consistency that's perfect for busy mornings or on-the-go breakfasts.

The beauty of overnight oats lies in their simplicity and nutritional profile. Oats are a whole grain rich in beta-glucan, a type of soluble fiber that has been shown to help lower cholesterol levels and improve heart health[13]. They're also a good source of complex carbohydrates, providing sustained energy throughout the morning. By preparing your oats the night before, you're not only saving time in the morning but also allowing the oats to soften and absorb the flavors of your chosen ingredients, resulting in a more digestible and flavorful breakfast.

The basic formula for overnight oats is simple:

- *1/2* cup rolled oats
- *1/2* cup liquid (milk, plant-based milk, or water)
- *1/4* cup yogurt (optional, for extra creaminess and protein)

- *1-2* tablespoons of mix-ins (chia seeds, nuts, dried fruit)
- Sweetener to taste (honey, maple syrup, or mashed banana)

One of the key advantages of overnight oats is their adaptability to various dietary needs and preferences. For those following a plant-based diet, using non-dairy milk and plant-based yogurt alternatives works perfectly. If you're looking to increase your protein intake, adding a scoop of protein powder or using Greek yogurt can boost the protein content significantly. For those watching their sugar intake, using mashed banana or unsweetened applesauce as a natural sweetener can be a great alternative to added sugars.

Let's explore some versatile overnight oats recipes to inspire your breakfast creations:

1. Classic Vanilla Berry Overnight Oats:

- *1/2* cup rolled oats
- *1/2* cup unsweetened almond milk
- *1/4* cup Greek yogurt
- *1* tablespoon chia seeds
- *1/2* teaspoon vanilla extract
- *1* tablespoon honey
- *1/4* cup mixed berries (fresh or frozen)

2. Chocolate Peanut Butter Banana Overnight Oats:

- *1/2* cup rolled oats
- *1/2* cup unsweetened almond milk
- *1* tablespoon unsweetened cocoa powder
- *1* tablespoon peanut butter
- *1/2* mashed banana
- *1* tablespoon maple syrup
- *1* tablespoon chopped peanuts (for topping)

3. Green Apple Pie Overnight Oats:

- *1/2* cup rolled oats
- *1/2* cup unsweetened almond milk
- *1/4* cup Greek yogurt
- *1/4* cup grated green apple
- *1/4* teaspoon cinnamon
- *1* tablespoon chopped walnuts
- *1* tablespoon maple syrup

When preparing your overnight oats, consider the texture you prefer. If you like your oats more liquid, add a bit more milk. For a thicker consistency, use less liquid or add more oats. The beauty of this method is that you can easily adjust the recipe to suit your preferences.

To add nutritional variety to your overnight oats, consider incorporating some of these nutrient-dense add-ins:

- Chia seeds or ground flaxseed for omega-3 fatty acids and additional fiber
- Protein powder for an extra protein boost
- Grated zucchini or carrots for added vegetables and fiber
- Pumpkin puree for vitamin A and fiber
- Cocoa powder for antioxidants and a chocolate flavor
- Matcha powder for antioxidants and a gentle caffeine boost

Overnight oats can be stored in the refrigerator for up to *5* days, making them an excellent option for meal prep. Prepare a batch at the beginning of the week, and you'll have breakfast ready to go for several days. If you prefer your oats warm, simply heat them in the microwave for *30-60* seconds before adding your toppings.

Remember, the key to enjoying overnight oats regularly is to keep experimenting with flavors and textures. Don't be afraid to try new combinations or to adapt your favorite dessert flavors into a healthier breakfast option. By mastering the art of overnight oats, you're equipping yourself with a versatile, nutritious breakfast option that can be tailored to your tastes and nutritional needs, ensuring that you start each day with a satisfying and energizing meal.

Savory Breakfast Options

While sweet breakfast options are popular, savory breakfasts offer a delicious and often overlooked alternative that can provide a diverse range of nutrients to start your day. Savory breakfasts tend to be rich in protein and vegetables, which can help keep you feeling full and satisfied throughout the morning. They also offer an excellent opportunity to incorporate more vegetables into your diet, contributing to your daily nutrient intake right from the start of the day.

Savory breakfasts can be particularly beneficial for those looking to manage their blood sugar levels or reduce their intake of added sugars. By focusing on protein, healthy fats, and complex carbohydrates, savory breakfast options can provide sustained energy and help prevent mid-morning energy crashes that are often associated with high-sugar breakfast choices.

Let's explore some nutritious and delicious savory breakfast ideas that you can incorporate into your morning routine:

1. Vegetable-Packed Frittata: A frittata is a versatile egg-based dish that can be customized with various vegetables and proteins. Here's a basic recipe:

- *6* large eggs
- *1/4* cup milk (dairy or plant-based)
- *1* cup mixed vegetables (e.g., spinach, bell peppers, onions)
- *1/4* cup crumbled feta cheese
- Salt and pepper to taste

2. Avocado Toast with Poached Egg: This popular breakfast option is both nutritious and satisfying:

- *1* slice of whole grain bread
- *1/2* ripe avocado

- *1* poached egg
- Cherry tomatoes, sliced
- Red pepper flakes and salt to taste

3. Savory Oatmeal Bowl: For a twist on traditional oatmeal, try this savory version:

- *1/2* cup rolled oats
- *1* cup vegetable broth
- *1/4* cup grated cheese (optional)
- *1* handful of baby spinach
- *1* soft-boiled egg
- Sliced green onions and sesame seeds for topping

4. Breakfast Burrito Bowl: A deconstructed burrito bowl can be a nutritious and filling breakfast option:

- *1/2* cup cooked quinoa or brown rice
- *1/4* cup black beans
- Scrambled eggs (*2* eggs)
- Diced tomatoes and avocado
- Handful of spinach or mixed greens
- Salsa and a dollop of Greek yogurt

5. Smoked Salmon and Cucumber Toast: For a protein-rich, omega-*3* packed breakfast, try this simple yet elegant option:

- *1* slice of whole grain bread
- *2* tablespoons cream cheese (or dairy-free alternative)
- *2* ounces smoked salmon
- Thinly sliced cucumber

- Capers and dill for garnish

When incorporating savory breakfasts into your routine, consider the following tips:

- Prep ingredients in advance: Chop vegetables, cook grains, or hard-boil eggs at the beginning of the week to make morning assembly quicker.
- Balance your plate: Aim to include a source of protein, complex carbohydrates, and vegetables in your savory breakfast for optimal nutrition and satiety.
- Experiment with herbs and spices: These can add flavor without extra calories and often come with their own health benefits.
- Don't forget about leftovers: Last night's roasted vegetables or grains can easily be repurposed into a nutritious savory breakfast.

Savory breakfasts offer an excellent opportunity to diversify your morning meal and increase your intake of vegetables and protein. By thinking outside the traditional breakfast box, you can create satisfying, nutrient-dense meals that fuel your body and mind for the day ahead. Whether you prefer a hearty frittata, a simple avocado toast, or a more elaborate breakfast bowl, there are countless ways to enjoy a savory start to your day.

Quick and Healthy Breakfast Ideas

In our fast-paced world, finding time for a nutritious breakfast can often feel challenging. However, a quick breakfast doesn't have to mean sacrificing nutrition. With a bit of planning and some creative ideas, you can enjoy a healthy, energizing breakfast even on your busiest mornings. This section will explore a variety of quick and easy breakfast options that are not only nutritious but also delicious and satisfying.

The key to successful quick breakfasts is preparation and having a repertoire of go-to recipes that can be assembled or reheated in minutes. By stocking your kitchen with versatile, nutrient-dense ingredients, you'll always have the building blocks for a healthy breakfast on hand. Let's explore some quick and healthy breakfast ideas that can be prepared in *10* minutes or less:

1. Yogurt Parfait: Layer Greek yogurt with fresh berries and a sprinkle of granola for a quick, protein-rich breakfast. Prepare the layers in a jar the night before for an easy grab-and-go option.

- *1* cup Greek yogurt
- *1/2* cup mixed berries
- *2* tablespoons low-sugar granola
- *1* teaspoon honey (optional)

2. Chia Seed Pudding: Prepare this the night before for a no-fuss morning meal.

- *2* tablespoons chia seeds
- *1/2* cup unsweetened almond milk
- *1/2* teaspoon vanilla extract
- *1* teaspoon maple syrup
- Toppings: sliced almonds and fresh fruit

3. Microwave Egg Scramble: For a warm, protein-packed breakfast in minutes:

- *2* eggs
- *1* handful of spinach
- *1* tablespoon milk
- *2* tablespoons shredded cheese
- Salt and pepper to taste

4. Whole Grain Toast with Toppings: Toast is a versatile base for quick, nutritious breakfasts. Try these combinations:

- Peanut butter and banana slices
- Mashed avocado with a sprinkle of everything bagel seasoning
- Hummus with sliced cucumber and tomato

5. Breakfast Smoothie: For a portable breakfast, blend:

- *1* cup unsweetened almond milk
- *1* frozen banana
- *1* tablespoon almond butter
- *1* handful of spinach
- *1* scoop protein powder (optional)
- *1/2* teaspoon cinnamon

6. Overnight Oats: Prepare these the night before for a ready-to-eat breakfast:

- *1/2* cup rolled oats
- *1/2* cup milk of choice
- *1/4* cup Greek yogurt
- *1* tablespoon chia seeds
- *1* tablespoon maple syrup
- *1/4* cup diced apple

7. Breakfast Quesadilla: For a savory, portable option:

- *1* whole wheat tortilla
- *1* scrambled egg
- *2* tablespoons black beans
- *2* tablespoons shredded cheese
- Salsa for dipping

To make quick, healthy breakfasts a regular part of your routine, consider these strategies:

- Prep ingredients in advance: Wash and chop fruits and vegetables, portion out dry ingredients, or cook grains in bulk at the beginning of the week.

- Stock your pantry and fridge with versatile, healthy ingredients: Keep items like Greek yogurt, eggs, whole grain bread, nut butters, and frozen fruits on hand.
- Invest in time-saving tools: A good blender for smoothies or a mini food processor for quick chopping can make breakfast prep much faster.
- Plan ahead: Take a few minutes each evening to think about what you'll have for breakfast the next day and do any necessary prep work.
- Repurpose leftovers: Last night's roasted vegetables or cooked grains can easily be incorporated into a quick breakfast scramble or bowl.

Remember, the goal is to start your day with a nutritious meal that will fuel your body and mind. Even a simple combination of a piece of fruit with a handful of nuts can be a better choice than skipping breakfast altogether. By having a variety of quick and easy options at your disposal, you'll be more likely to make time for this important meal, setting a positive tone for the rest of your day.

Quick and healthy breakfasts don't have to be complicated or time-consuming. With a little planning and creativity, you can enjoy nutritious, delicious breakfasts that fit into even the busiest of schedules. By prioritizing your morning meal, you're making an investment in your health and well-being, providing your body with the fuel it needs to tackle whatever the day may bring.

Chapter 7: Satisfying Lunch Recipes

Lunch is a crucial meal that can set the tone for the rest of your day. A well-balanced, nutritious lunch not only satisfies your hunger but also provides the energy and nutrients needed to power through afternoon activities. In this chapter, we'll explore a variety of delicious and healthy lunch options that are easy to prepare, packed with nutrients, and adaptable to different tastes and dietary needs. From vibrant salads to hearty grain bowls, comforting soups to convenient wraps, you'll discover a wealth of recipes and ideas to keep your midday meals exciting and nourishing.

The key to a satisfying lunch lies in balancing macronutrients, incorporating a variety of vegetables, and choosing ingredients that provide sustained energy. We'll focus on recipes that combine complex carbohydrates, lean proteins, and healthy fats to create meals that keep you full and focused throughout the afternoon. Additionally, we'll explore ways to make these lunches portable and convenient for those who need to eat on-the-go or at their workplace.

As we delve into each category of lunch recipes, you'll learn not only how to prepare these dishes but also how to customize them to suit your preferences and nutritional needs. We'll discuss the benefits of each ingredient, provide tips for meal prep, and offer suggestions for variations to keep your lunch routine fresh and exciting. Whether you're looking to incorporate more plant-based meals into your diet, increase your vegetable intake, or simply find new ways to enjoy healthy eating, this chapter will provide you with the inspiration and knowledge to create lunches that are both nutritious and delicious.

Power-Packed Salads

Salads have come a long way from the bland, uninspiring bowls of iceberg lettuce and a few token vegetables. Today's power salads are nutrient-dense, flavor-packed meals that can easily stand alone as a satisfying lunch. The key to creating a power salad lies in combining a variety of ingredients that offer a balance of nutrients, textures, and flavors. Start with a base of leafy greens, which provide fiber, vitamins, and minerals. Dark, leafy greens like spinach, kale, and arugula are particularly nutrient-rich choices. To this base, add a mix of colorful vegetables to increase the nutritional value and visual appeal of your salad. Think beyond the usual suspects and incorporate roasted vegetables, grilled zucchini, or shredded Brussels sprouts for added depth and flavor.

Protein is an essential component of a power salad, helping to keep you full and satisfied throughout the afternoon. Lean proteins such as grilled chicken, hard-boiled eggs, or canned tuna are excellent options. For plant-based alternatives, consider adding chickpeas, lentils, or tofu. These protein sources not only contribute to the satiety factor of your salad but also provide essential amino acids necessary for various bodily functions. To round out your power salad, include a source of healthy fats. Avocado, nuts, seeds, or a drizzle of olive oil can add richness and help your body absorb fat-soluble vitamins from the vegetables.

One of the advantages of power salads is their versatility. You can easily adapt them to use seasonal produce, accommodate dietary restrictions, or simply cater to your taste preferences. For example, a summer salad might feature fresh berries and grilled peaches, while an autumn salad could incorporate roasted squash and crisp apples. Experiment with different combinations to keep your lunches interesting and take advantage of the best produce available throughout the year.

When it comes to dressing your power salad, opt for homemade vinaigrettes or light dressings that complement the flavors of your ingredients without overwhelming them. A simple combination of olive oil, lemon juice, and herbs can be just as delicious as more complex dressings and allows the natural flavors of your salad ingredients to shine. If you're preparing your salad in advance, consider packing the dressing separately to prevent the greens from becoming soggy.

Here's a recipe for a Mediterranean-inspired power salad that exemplifies the principles we've discussed:

- *2* cups mixed greens (spinach, arugula, and romaine)
- *1/2* cup cherry tomatoes, halved
- *1/4* cup cucumber, diced
- *1/4* cup red onion, thinly sliced
- *1/4* cup kalamata olives, pitted and halved
- *1/4* cup feta cheese, crumbled

- *1/2* cup cooked quinoa
- *4* oz grilled chicken breast, sliced
- *1/4* avocado, sliced
- *2* tablespoons toasted pine nuts
- Lemon-herb vinaigrette (*2* tablespoons olive oil, *1* tablespoon lemon juice, *1* teaspoon Dijon mustard, *1* teaspoon honey, *1* tablespoon chopped fresh herbs like parsley and oregano, salt and pepper to taste)

Remember, the key to making power salads a regular part of your lunch routine is preparation. Consider batch-cooking ingredients like grilled chicken, roasted vegetables, and grains at the beginning of the week. Store these components separately in the refrigerator, and you'll be able to quickly assemble fresh, varied salads throughout the week. This approach not only saves time but also ensures that you have healthy, homemade lunches ready to go, reducing the temptation to opt for less nutritious convenience foods.

Balanced Grain Bowls

Grain bowls have become increasingly popular in recent years, and for good reason. These versatile, nutrient-dense meals offer a perfect balance of complex carbohydrates, proteins, and healthy fats, making them an ideal choice for a satisfying and energizing lunch. The foundation of a grain bowl is, as the name suggests, a serving of whole grains. Options like quinoa, brown rice, farro, or barley provide a hearty base that's rich in fiber and *B* vitamins. These complex carbohydrates offer sustained energy release, helping to keep you full and focused throughout the afternoon.

Building a balanced grain bowl is an art that combines nutrition science with culinary creativity. Start by choosing your grain base, then layer on a variety of colorful vegetables. Raw, roasted, or grilled vegetables can all work well, adding different textures and flavors to your bowl. Aim for a rainbow of colors to ensure you're getting a wide range of vitamins, minerals, and antioxidants. Next, add a source of protein to make your grain bowl more satiating and complete. This could be plant-based options like chickpeas, lentils, or tofu, or animal proteins such as grilled chicken, salmon, or a hard-boiled egg.

To elevate your grain bowl from good to great, consider adding elements that provide contrasting textures and flavors. A sprinkle of nuts or seeds can add crunch and healthy fats. Fresh herbs bring brightness and additional nutrients. A dollop of hummus or a drizzle of tahini sauce can add creaminess and depth of flavor. Finally, don't forget about the dressing. A well-crafted dressing can tie all the elements of your grain bowl together, enhancing the overall taste experience.

One of the advantages of grain bowls is their adaptability to different cuisines and flavor profiles. You can create a Mediterranean-inspired bowl with quinoa, roasted vegetables, feta cheese, and a lemon-herb dressing. Or, opt for an Asian-inspired version with brown rice, edamame, pickled vegetables, and a miso-ginger dressing. The possibilities are virtually endless, allowing you to keep your lunches varied and exciting.

Here's a recipe for a nourishing autumn grain bowl that showcases seasonal ingredients:

- *1/2* cup cooked farro
- *1* cup roasted butternut squash cubes
- *1/2* cup massaged kale
- *1/4* cup pomegranate seeds
- *2* tablespoons crumbled goat cheese
- *2* tablespoons toasted pumpkin seeds
- *2* oz grilled chicken breast, sliced (optional)
- Apple cider vinaigrette (*1* tablespoon apple cider vinegar, *2* tablespoons olive oil, *1* teaspoon Dijon mustard, *1* teaspoon maple syrup, salt and pepper to taste)

When preparing grain bowls for lunch, consider the concept of batch cooking to streamline your meal prep. Cook a large quantity of grains and roast a variety of vegetables at the beginning of the week. Store these components separately in the refrigerator, and you can easily assemble fresh bowls throughout the week. This approach not only saves time but also allows for variety in your lunches, as you can mix and match different components each day.

Remember that while grains form the base of these bowls, they shouldn't dominate the meal. Aim for a balance where vegetables make up the largest portion of your bowl, followed by protein, then grains. This ensures you're getting a nutrient-dense meal that aligns with healthy eating guidelines. By mastering the art of the balanced grain bowl, you'll have a versatile, satisfying lunch option that can be adapted to suit your tastes and nutritional needs throughout the year.

Nourishing Soups and Stews

Soups and stews are often overlooked as lunch options, but they can be some of the most nourishing and satisfying meals to enjoy midday. These one-pot wonders are not only comforting but also offer an excellent opportunity to pack a variety of nutrients into a single dish. From light, broth-based soups to hearty, vegetable-packed stews, there's a wide range of options to suit different tastes and nutritional needs. What makes soups and stews particularly beneficial for lunch is their ability to provide hydration along with sustenance, helping you feel satisfied and energized for the rest of the day.

When crafting a nutritious soup or stew for lunch, start with a base of vegetables. This could be a classic mirepoix of onions, carrots, and celery, or a more diverse mix including leafy greens, root vegetables, or squash. The vegetables provide fiber, vitamins, and minerals, forming the nutritional foundation of your meal. Next, consider your protein source. This could be plant-based options like beans or lentils, which also contribute additional fiber, or lean animal proteins like chicken or fish. The protein helps to make your soup more satiating and supports muscle health and repair.

The liquid base of your soup or stew is another opportunity to boost nutrition. While water is always an option, using homemade or low-sodium broths can add depth of flavor and additional nutrients. Bone broth, for instance, provides collagen and amino acids that support gut health and joint function. For creamy soups, consider using pureed vegetables or legumes as a base instead of heavy cream. This not only reduces the calorie content but also increases the fiber and nutrient density of your soup.

Herbs and spices play a crucial role in elevating the flavor profile of soups and stews while also contributing additional health benefits. Turmeric, for example, has anti-inflammatory properties, while garlic and ginger can support immune function. Don't be afraid to experiment with different herb and spice combinations to create unique and flavorful soups.

Here's a recipe for a nutrient-dense lentil and vegetable soup that's perfect for a satisfying lunch:

- *1* cup dried green or brown lentils, rinsed
- *1* onion, diced
- *2* carrots, diced
- *2* celery stalks, diced
- *2* cloves garlic, minced
- *1* can (*14.5* oz) diced tomatoes
- *4* cups low-sodium vegetable broth
- *2* cups chopped kale
- *1* tablespoon olive oil
- *1* teaspoon ground cumin
- *1* teaspoon smoked paprika
- Salt and pepper to taste
- Juice of *1* lemon

One of the great advantages of soups and stews for lunch is their make-ahead potential. Many soups actually improve in flavor after a day or two, as the ingredients have time to meld together. Consider making a large batch of soup at the beginning of the week and portioning it out for several lunches. This not only saves time but also ensures you have a nutritious meal ready to go, reducing the temptation to opt for less healthy convenience foods.

When packing soup for lunch, invest in a good quality, insulated container to keep your soup hot until lunchtime. If your soup is particularly thick or stew-like, you might want to pack some additional broth separately to thin it out if needed when reheating. Don't forget to include some whole grain bread or crackers on the side for added texture and to help round out the meal.

Remember that soups and stews can be easily adapted to suit different dietary needs and preferences. For a lower-carb option, focus on vegetable-based soups with lean proteins. For those following a plant-based diet, legume and vegetable soups can provide complete nutrition. By mastering the art of soup and stew making, you'll have a versatile, comforting, and nutritious option for lunches throughout the year, particularly welcome during cooler months.

Healthy Wraps and Sandwiches

Wraps and sandwiches are lunchtime staples for good reason - they're portable, customizable, and can be packed with a variety of nutritious ingredients. However, not all wraps and sandwiches are created equal when it comes to health and nutrition. The key to creating a healthy wrap or sandwich lies in choosing wholesome ingredients and maintaining a balance of nutrients. When done right, these handheld meals can provide a perfect combination of complex carbohydrates, lean proteins, healthy fats, and plenty of vegetables, offering a satisfying and nutritious lunch option.

The foundation of any healthy wrap or sandwich is the bread or wrap itself. Opt for whole grain options which provide more fiber, vitamins, and minerals compared to their refined counterparts. Whole grain breads, wraps, or even lettuce leaves can serve as an excellent base. If using bread, choose varieties with minimal added sugars and preservatives. For those watching their carbohydrate intake, consider using a single slice of bread to make an open-faced sandwich, or use large lettuce leaves as a wrap alternative.

Next, focus on adding a lean protein source. This could be sliced turkey or chicken breast, canned tuna or salmon, hard-boiled eggs, or plant-based options like hummus, tofu, or tempeh. Protein is crucial for keeping you feeling full and satisfied throughout the afternoon. Aim for about 3-4 ounces of protein per sandwich or wrap. Remember that if you're using a plant-based protein, you may need to increase the quantity slightly to match the protein content of animal-based options.

Vegetables are where you can really boost the nutritional value of your wrap or sandwich. Don't limit yourself to just lettuce and tomato - consider adding cucumber slices, shredded carrots, roasted red peppers, spinach leaves, or sprouts. These not only add vitamins, minerals, and fiber but also provide a variety of textures and flavors. Aim to include at least two different vegetables in your wrap or sandwich.

Here's a recipe for a nutrient-packed Mediterranean Veggie Wrap that exemplifies these principles:

- *1* whole grain wrap
- *2* tablespoons hummus
- *1/4* cup mixed salad greens
- *1/4* cup cucumber, thinly sliced

- *1/4* cup roasted red peppers, sliced
- *2* tablespoons crumbled feta cheese
- *5-6* kalamata olives, pitted and sliced
- *1* tablespoon sunflower seeds
- *1* teaspoon olive oil
- *1* teaspoon lemon juice
- Pinch of dried oregano

When it comes to condiments and spreads, choose options that add flavor without excessive calories or unhealthy fats. Mustard, hummus, mashed avocado, or a small amount of olive oil-based dressing can enhance the taste of your wrap or sandwich while contributing beneficial nutrients. Be cautious with mayonnaise, cheese, and high-sugar spreads, using them sparingly if at all.

For those who prefer traditional sandwiches, consider this formula for a balanced, nutritious option: Start with two slices of whole grain bread. Add *3-4* ounces of lean protein (such as turkey breast or mashed chickpeas), a serving of healthy fat (like avocado or a thin spread of nut butter), and pile on the vegetables (lettuce, tomato, cucumber, sprouts). If desired, add a slice of cheese or a spread like hummus for additional flavor and nutrients.

One of the advantages of wraps and sandwiches is their portability. They're easy to pack and take with you to work or on-the-go. To keep your wrap or sandwich fresh until lunchtime, consider packing wet ingredients like tomatoes separately and adding them just before eating. If using lettuce or other leafy greens, wrap them in a paper towel to absorb excess moisture and keep them crisp.

Remember that variety is key to maintaining a healthy and interesting lunch routine. Rotate different types of wraps, breads, proteins, and vegetables to keep your meals exciting and ensure you're getting a wide range of nutrients. By mastering the art of creating healthy wraps and sandwiches, you'll have a quick, easy, and nutritious lunch option that can be adapted to suit your tastes and nutritional needs throughout the week.

Chapter 8: Nourishing Dinner Recipes

Dinner is often considered the cornerstone of daily nutrition, providing an opportunity to replenish and nourish your body after a long day. This chapter delves into a variety of nourishing dinner recipes that not only satisfy your taste buds but also provide essential nutrients to support your overall health. By incorporating these recipes into your meal rotation, you'll discover how easy and enjoyable it can be to create wholesome, delicious dinners that align with your health goals.

The recipes in this chapter are designed to be versatile, allowing you to adapt them to your preferences and dietary needs. Whether you're looking to increase your plant-based intake, incorporate more lean proteins, or simply want to explore new flavors, these recipes offer something for everyone. Each recipe is carefully crafted to ensure a balance of nutrients, flavors, and textures, making your dinner not just a meal, but an experience to look forward to.

As you explore these recipes, remember that cooking is both an art and a science. Feel free to experiment with different ingredients or cooking methods to suit your taste. The key is to maintain nutritional balance while allowing your creativity to shine through. Let's embark on this culinary journey to transform your dinner routine into a nourishing and enjoyable part of your day.

Flavorful Plant-Based Main Courses

Plant-based main courses have gained popularity not only for their health benefits but also for their incredible flavor potential. These dishes prove that vegetarian and vegan meals can be just as satisfying and protein-rich as their meat-based counterparts. By focusing on whole plant foods, you can create meals that are high in fiber, vitamins, minerals, and antioxidants, while also being environmentally sustainable.

One standout recipe in this category is the Quinoa-Stuffed Bell Peppers. This dish combines protein-rich quinoa with a medley of vegetables, herbs, and spices, all nestled in colorful bell peppers. To prepare, start by cooking quinoa according to package instructions, then sauté onions, garlic, and your choice of diced vegetables (such as zucchini, carrots, and mushrooms) in olive oil. Mix the sautéed vegetables with the cooked quinoa, adding herbs like parsley and mint for freshness. Cut bell peppers in half, remove the seeds, and stuff them with the quinoa mixture. Bake in the oven at *375°F (190°C)* for about *25-30* minutes until the peppers are tender. This dish not only looks impressive but also provides a complete protein source when quinoa is combined with vegetables.

Another delightful plant-based option is the Lentil and Sweet Potato Curry. This hearty dish is packed with flavor and nutrition. Begin by sautéing onions, garlic, and ginger in a large pot. Add curry powder, turmeric, and cumin for a fragrant base. Next, add diced sweet potatoes, red lentils, and vegetable broth. Simmer until the lentils and sweet potatoes are tender, about *20-25* minutes. Finish with a can of coconut milk for creaminess and a handful of spinach for added nutrients. This curry is not only rich in protein from the lentils but also provides complex carbohydrates from the sweet potatoes and a wealth of vitamins and minerals from the various spices and vegetables.

For those looking for a meat-like texture in their plant-based meals, consider trying a Portobello Mushroom Steak. Marinate large portobello mushroom caps in a mixture of balsamic vinegar, soy sauce, garlic, and herbs for at least *30* minutes. Grill or pan-sear the mushrooms until they're tender and have nice grill marks. Serve with a side of roasted vegetables and quinoa or brown rice for a complete meal. Portobello mushrooms are not only low in calories but also provide a good amount of selenium, potassium, and *B* vitamins.

Incorporating legumes into your plant-based main courses is an excellent way to ensure you're getting enough protein. A Chickpea and Spinach Stew is a perfect example of how legumes can form the basis of a satisfying meal. Start by sautéing onions and garlic, then add diced tomatoes, chickpeas, and vegetable broth. Season with cumin, paprika, and a touch of cinnamon for depth of flavor. Simmer until the chickpeas are tender, then stir in a large handful of fresh spinach just before serving. This stew is not only rich in protein and fiber from the chickpeas but also provides iron and vitamins *A* and *C* from the spinach.

For a refreshing summer dinner, try a Buddha Bowl filled with a variety of colorful vegetables, grains, and plant-based proteins. Start with a base of quinoa or brown rice, then add roasted vegetables like sweet potatoes, broccoli, and bell peppers. Include a protein source such as edamame or crispy baked tofu. Top with sliced avocado, a sprinkle of seeds (like pumpkin or sunflower seeds), and a drizzle of tahini dressing. Buddha Bowls are not only visually appealing but also offer a balanced meal with a variety of nutrients from different food groups.

Remember, the key to creating satisfying plant-based main courses is to focus on a variety of textures, colors, and flavors. Don't be afraid to experiment with different plant proteins like tempeh, seitan, or various legumes. By incorporating a wide range of plant-based ingredients, you ensure that your meals are not only delicious but also nutritionally diverse, providing your body with the full spectrum of nutrients it needs to thrive.

Lean Protein Dishes

Lean protein dishes are essential for maintaining muscle mass, supporting metabolic health, and promoting satiety. These recipes focus on incorporating high-quality proteins while keeping overall fat content in check. By choosing lean proteins, you can enjoy flavorful meals that support your health goals without sacrificing taste or satisfaction.

One excellent lean protein option is Grilled Lemon Herb Chicken Breast. Start by marinating chicken breasts in a mixture of lemon juice, olive oil, garlic, and a blend of herbs like rosemary, thyme, and oregano for at least *30* minutes. Grill the chicken over medium-high heat for about 6-8 minutes per side, or until the internal temperature reaches *165°F* (*74°C*). This cooking method allows excess fat to drip away while the chicken cooks, resulting in a leaner dish. Serve with a side of grilled vegetables and quinoa for a complete meal. Chicken breast is an excellent source of lean protein, providing about *31* grams of protein per *100*-gram serving, while being low in saturated fat[14].

For seafood lovers, Baked Salmon with Dill and Lemon is a nutrient-dense option. Preheat your oven to *400°F* (*200°C*). Place salmon fillets on a baking sheet lined with parchment paper. Drizzle with olive oil and sprinkle with fresh dill, lemon zest, salt, and pepper. Bake for about *12-15* minutes, depending on the thickness of the fillets. Salmon is not only rich in high-quality protein but also provides omega-*3* fatty acids, which are essential for heart and brain health[15].

A vegetarian option that's high in protein is Tofu Stir-Fry with Mixed Vegetables. Start by pressing firm tofu to remove excess moisture, then cut it into cubes. In a wok or large skillet, stir-fry the tofu in a small amount of oil until golden brown. Remove the tofu and set aside. In the same pan, stir-fry a variety of colorful vegetables like bell peppers, broccoli, carrots, and snap peas. Add minced garlic and ginger for flavor. Return the tofu to the pan and toss everything with a sauce made from low-sodium soy sauce, rice vinegar, and a touch of honey. Serve over brown rice or cauliflower rice. Tofu is an excellent plant-based protein source, providing all essential amino acids and being naturally low in saturated fat[16].

For a lean red meat option, consider Grilled Sirloin Steak with Chimichurri Sauce. Choose a lean cut of sirloin and trim any visible fat. Season the steak with salt and pepper, then grill to your desired doneness. While the steak is resting, prepare the chimichurri sauce by blending fresh parsley, cilantro, garlic, red wine vinegar, olive oil, and a pinch of red pepper flakes. Slice the steak thinly against the grain and serve with the chimichurri sauce on top. Pair with roasted sweet potato wedges and a mixed green salad. Lean beef sirloin provides high-quality protein along with important nutrients like iron and vitamin *B12*[17].

Egg-based dishes can also be excellent sources of lean protein. A Vegetable Frittata is a versatile option that can be customized based on your preferences. Whisk together eggs with a splash of milk, salt, and pepper. In an oven-safe skillet, sauté your choice of vegetables (such as spinach, mushrooms, and cherry tomatoes) in a small amount of olive oil. Pour the egg mixture over the vegetables and cook on the stovetop until the edges start to set. Transfer the skillet to a preheated oven and bake at *375°F* (*190°C*) for about *10-15* minutes, or until the frittata is fully set and lightly golden on top. Eggs are not only rich in high-quality protein but also provide essential nutrients like choline, which is important for brain health[18].

When preparing lean protein dishes, it's important to focus on cooking methods that don't add unnecessary fats. Grilling, baking, roasting, and steaming are excellent options that allow the natural flavors of the protein to shine through without adding extra calories. Additionally, pairing lean proteins with a variety of vegetables and whole grains ensures a well-balanced meal that provides a full spectrum of nutrients. By incorporating these lean protein dishes into your dinner rotation, you can enjoy satisfying meals that support your health and fitness goals.

Nutritious One-Pot Meals

One-pot meals are a game-winner for busy individuals looking to prepare nutritious dinners with minimal fuss and cleanup. These dishes combine proteins, vegetables, and often grains or legumes in a single cooking vessel, resulting in flavorful, well-balanced meals. The beauty of one-pot cooking lies not only in its convenience but also in how the flavors meld together during the cooking process, creating rich, satisfying dishes.

A classic one-pot meal is the Hearty Vegetable and Bean Soup. Start by sautéing onions, carrots, and celery in a large pot with a bit of olive oil. Add minced garlic and your choice of herbs like thyme and rosemary. Pour in low-sodium vegetable broth and add diced tomatoes, a variety of chopped vegetables (such as zucchini, green beans, and bell peppers), and your choice of beans (like cannellini or kidney beans). Simmer for about *20-25* minutes until the vegetables are tender. Finish with a handful of chopped kale or spinach for added nutrients. This soup is not only rich in fiber and plant-based protein from the beans but also provides a wide array of vitamins and minerals from the diverse vegetable content.

Another excellent one-pot option is the Mediterranean Chicken and Quinoa Skillet. In a large skillet, brown chicken pieces seasoned with Herbs de Provence. Remove the chicken and in the same pan, sauté onions, garlic, and bell peppers. Add quinoa and chicken broth, then nestle the chicken pieces back into the pan. Cover and simmer until the quinoa is cooked and the chicken is tender, about *20* minutes. Stir in halved cherry tomatoes, olives, and crumbled feta cheese at the end. This dish combines lean protein from the chicken with whole grain quinoa and a variety of vegetables, creating a balanced meal rich in Mediterranean flavors.

For a plant-based one-pot meal, try a Lentil and Vegetable Curry. In a large pot, sauté onions, garlic, and ginger. Add curry powder, turmeric, and cumin, then stir in red lentils, diced sweet potatoes, and vegetable broth. Simmer until the lentils and sweet potatoes are tender, about *20* minutes. Add a can of coconut milk and a variety of chopped vegetables like cauliflower, bell peppers, and spinach. Cook for an additional *5-10* minutes until the vegetables are tender-crisp. This curry is not only rich in plant-based protein and fiber from the lentils but also provides a wealth of antioxidants from the spices and vegetables.

A comforting one-pot option is the Turkey and Vegetable Quinoa Casserole. Brown ground turkey in a large oven-safe pot or Dutch oven. Add diced onions, carrots, and celery, cooking until softened. Stir in quinoa, diced tomatoes, and chicken broth. Bring to a simmer, then cover and transfer to a preheated oven. Bake at *375°F (190°C)* for about *25-30* minutes, or until the quinoa is cooked and most of the liquid is absorbed. Stir in frozen peas and top with shredded cheese before serving. This casserole provides a balance of lean protein, whole grains, and vegetables in a single dish.

For seafood lovers, a One-Pot Shrimp and Whole Grain Rice Pilaf is a delicious option. In a large pot, sauté onions and garlic, then add whole grain rice (such as brown rice or a wild rice blend) and toast it briefly. Pour in seafood or vegetable broth and bring to a simmer. Cover and cook until the rice is nearly tender, about *35-40* minutes. Stir in peeled shrimp and peas, cover, and cook for an additional *5-7* minutes until the shrimp are pink and cooked through. Finish with a squeeze of lemon juice and chopped fresh herbs. This dish combines lean protein from the shrimp with fiber-rich whole grains and vegetables, creating a well-rounded meal.

When preparing one-pot meals, it's important to layer flavors and textures to create satisfying dishes. Start with aromatic ingredients like onions and garlic as a flavor base, then build upon that with herbs, spices, and a variety of vegetables. Choose ingredients with different cooking times, adding quicker-cooking items towards the end to prevent overcooking. By mastering the art of one-pot cooking, you can create nutritious, delicious meals with minimal effort and cleanup, making it easier to maintain healthy eating habits even on busy weeknights.

Creative Vegetable Side Dishes

Vegetable side dishes are an essential component of a balanced meal, providing vital nutrients, fiber, and a burst of color to your plate. By exploring creative ways to prepare vegetables, you can transform them from mere accompaniments to star attractions that complement and enhance your main course. These innovative side dishes not only boost the nutritional value of your meals but also add variety and excitement to your dinner table.

One delightful vegetable side dish is Roasted Rainbow Carrots with Honey and Thyme. Start by washing and trimming a bunch of multi-colored carrots, leaving a bit of the green tops for presentation. Toss the carrots with olive oil, honey, fresh thyme leaves, salt, and pepper. Spread them on a baking sheet and roast at *400°F* (*200°C*) for about *20-25* minutes, or until tender and caramelized. The natural sweetness of the carrots is enhanced by the honey, while the thyme adds a subtle earthy flavor. This dish not only looks stunning with its array of colors but also provides a good source of beta-carotene, fiber, and antioxidants[19].

For a unique twist on a classic vegetable, try Cauliflower 'Rice' Pilaf. Pulse cauliflower florets in a food processor until they resemble rice grains. In a large skillet, sauté minced onions and garlic in olive oil. Add the cauliflower 'rice' and cook for about *5-7* minutes until tender. Stir in toasted almonds, dried cranberries, chopped fresh parsley, and a squeeze of lemon juice. Season with salt and pepper to taste. This low-carb alternative to traditional rice pilaf is rich in vitamins *C* and *K* and provides a good amount of fiber[20].

A Mediterranean-inspired side dish is Grilled Zucchini with Lemon and Feta. Slice zucchini lengthwise into thin planks. Brush with olive oil and season with salt and pepper. Grill over medium-high heat for *2-3* minutes per side until tender and lightly charred. Arrange the grilled zucchini on a platter and drizzle with a mixture of lemon juice and olive oil. Top with crumbled feta cheese, chopped fresh mint, and a sprinkle of red pepper flakes. This dish is not only low in calories but also provides a good source of vitamins *A* and *C*, as well as potassium[21].

For a hearty and nutritious side, consider Roasted Brussels Sprouts with Balsamic Glaze and Pecans. Trim and halve Brussels sprouts, then toss with olive oil, salt, and pepper. Roast at *400°F* (*200°C*) for about *20-25* minutes, shaking the pan halfway through, until crispy on the outside and tender on the inside. While the Brussels sprouts are roasting, reduce balsamic vinegar in a small saucepan until syrupy. Drizzle the balsamic glaze over the roasted Brussels sprouts and top with toasted pecans. This dish is rich in vitamin *C*, fiber, and antioxidants, and the addition of pecans provides healthy fats and a satisfying crunch[22].

A colorful and nutrient-dense option is the Rainbow Vegetable Slaw. Using a mandoline or sharp knife, thinly slice red cabbage, carrots, bell peppers, and radishes. Toss the vegetables with a dressing made from Greek yogurt, apple cider vinegar, Dijon mustard, honey, and a pinch of celery seeds. Let the slaw sit for at least *30* minutes before serving to allow the flavors to meld. This vibrant side dish not only provides a satisfying crunch but also offers a wide array of vitamins, minerals, and antioxidants from the diverse vegetable content[23].

When creating vegetable side dishes, focus on enhancing the natural flavors of the vegetables while adding complementary tastes and textures. Experiment with different cooking methods such as roasting, grilling, or sautéing to bring out unique flavors. Don't be afraid to combine vegetables with fruits, nuts, or cheese for added interest and nutritional value. By incorporating a variety of colorful and creatively prepared vegetable sides into your meals, you can ensure that you're getting a wide range of nutrients while keeping your dinners exciting and satisfying.

Chapter 9: Healthy Snacks and Desserts

In the journey towards a healthier lifestyle, snacks and desserts often present a significant challenge. Many people associate these food categories with unhealthy options that can derail their nutritional goals. However, with the right approach and recipes, snacks and desserts can be both delicious and nutritious, supporting your overall health and well-being. This chapter will explore various ways to create satisfying snacks and indulgent desserts that align with your healthy eating habits.

The key to incorporating snacks and desserts into a healthy diet lies in understanding their role in your overall nutrition plan. Snacks can serve as mini-meals that help maintain stable blood sugar levels, provide sustained energy throughout the day, and prevent overeating during main meals. Desserts, when prepared with wholesome ingredients and consumed in moderation, can be a part of a balanced diet, satisfying your sweet tooth without compromising your health goals.

Throughout this chapter, you'll discover a variety of recipes and techniques for creating nutritious snacks and desserts. From no-bake energy bites that offer a quick and portable source of fuel to smart snacking options that keep you satisfied between meals; you'll learn how to make choices that support your health. We'll also explore fruit-based desserts that capitalize on nature's sweetness and healthier baking alternatives that allow you to enjoy your favorite treats with a nutritious twist.

As you explore these recipes and ideas, remember that the goal is not to deprive yourself of enjoyable foods but to find ways to nourish your body while still savoring the pleasures of eating. By incorporating these healthier snack and dessert options into your routine, you'll be better equipped to maintain a balanced diet that supports your overall health and well-being.

No-Bake Energy Bites

No-bake energy bites have gained popularity in recent years as a convenient, nutritious snack option. These small, portable treats are packed with wholesome ingredients that provide a quick energy boost without the need for baking. The beauty of energy bites lies in their versatility and ease of preparation, making them an excellent choice for busy individuals looking to maintain a healthy diet.

The foundation of most energy bite recipes typically includes a combination of nuts, seeds, dried fruits, and a binding agent such as nut butter or honey. This combination provides a balance of complex carbohydrates, healthy fats, and protein, which work together to offer sustained energy release. For example, a classic energy bite might contain rolled oats (complex carbs), almonds (protein and healthy fats), dates (natural sweetness and fiber), and almond butter (healthy fats and protein) as its core ingredients.

One of the key advantages of energy bites is their nutrient density. In just a small serving, you can pack a significant number of vitamins, minerals, and other beneficial compounds. For instance, adding chia seeds to your energy bites can boost their omega-*3* fatty acid content, while incorporating cacao powder can introduce antioxidants. This nutrient density makes energy bites an excellent option for pre- or post-workout snacks, mid-afternoon pick-me-ups, or even as a quick breakfast on busy mornings.

When creating your own energy bite recipes, it's important to consider the balance of flavors and textures. A good energy bite should have a pleasant mouthfeel and a taste that keeps you coming back for more. Experiment with different combinations of nuts and seeds for crunch, dried fruits for chewiness and natural sweetness, and spices like cinnamon or vanilla for added depth of flavor. You can also incorporate superfoods like goji berries, maca powder, or spirulina to boost the nutritional profile even further.

Here's a basic recipe to get you started:

- *1* cup rolled oats
- *1/2* cup nut butter of choice (e.g., almond, peanut, or cashew butter)
- *1/3* cup honey or maple syrup
- *1/4* cup ground flaxseed
- *1/4* cup mini dark chocolate chips
- *1* teaspoon vanilla extract

To keep your energy bites interesting and aligned with your nutritional goals, consider rotating ingredients based on what's available seasonally or what aligns with your current health focus.

For example, if you're looking to increase your intake of anti-inflammatory foods, you might incorporate turmeric and black pepper into a golden milk-inspired energy bite. If you're focusing on gut health, adding ingredients like ground flaxseed or chia seeds can boost the fiber content.

It's worth noting that while energy bites are a nutritious snack option, they are calorie-dense. This makes them excellent for providing quick energy, but it also means that portion control is important. Generally, one or two energy bites make for a satisfying snack. Be mindful of your overall daily calorie and nutrient intake when incorporating these into your diet.

For those with specific dietary requirements, energy bites can easily be adapted. For a vegan version, use maple syrup instead of honey. If you're following a gluten-free diet, ensure your oats are certified gluten-free. For nut allergies, sunflower seed butter can be an excellent alternative to nut butters.

In conclusion, no-bake energy bites offer a convenient, customizable, and nutritious snack option that can support your healthy eating goals. By experimenting with different ingredients and flavors, you can create a variety of energy bites that not only satisfy your taste buds but also provide the nutrients your body needs to thrive throughout the day.

Smart Snacking Options

Smart snacking is an essential component of a balanced and healthy diet. When done right, snacking can help maintain stable blood sugar levels, prevent overeating at main meals, and provide your body with a steady stream of nutrients throughout the day. The key to smart snacking lies in choosing nutrient-dense foods that satisfy hunger without compromising your overall nutritional goals.

One of the fundamental principles of smart snacking is to combine macronutrients. A snack that includes a mix of complex carbohydrates, lean proteins, and healthy fats will keep you feeling fuller for longer and provide sustained energy. For example, apple slices (carbohydrates) paired with almond butter (protein and healthy fats) create a balanced snack that offers both immediate and long-lasting energy.

Portion control is another crucial aspect of smart snacking. While snacks are meant to tide you over between meals, they shouldn't be so large that they replace a main meal. A good rule of thumb is to keep snacks between *150-250* calories, depending on your individual needs and activity level. Using small plates or pre-portioning snacks can help prevent mindless overeating.

Vegetables and fruits should form the foundation of many of your snacks. These foods are rich in vitamins, minerals, and fiber, while being relatively low in calories. Crunchy vegetables like carrots, celery, and bell peppers can satisfy the urge to snack while providing essential nutrients. Pairing these with a healthy dip like hummus or guacamole adds flavor and additional nutrients. Fruits, whether fresh, frozen, or dried (in moderation), offer natural sweetness and a host of beneficial compounds.

Protein-rich snacks are particularly effective for maintaining satiety. Greek yogurt, hard-boiled eggs, edamame, or a small handful of nuts are all excellent options. These foods not only help keep you full but also support muscle maintenance and growth. For those following a plant-based diet, options like roasted chickpeas or a small serving of quinoa salad can provide the necessary protein boost.

Whole grains should also feature in your snacking repertoire. They provide complex carbohydrates that offer sustained energy release. Whole grain crackers, air-popped popcorn, or a small serving of oatmeal can make for satisfying snacks. When choosing grain-based snacks, always opt for whole grain varieties to maximize nutrient intake and fiber content.

For those with a sweet tooth, it's important to find healthier alternatives to traditional sugary snacks. Dark chocolate (*70%* cocoa or higher) in moderation can satisfy cravings while providing antioxidants. Frozen grapes or banana slices can serve as a naturally sweet treat. Chia seed pudding made with unsweetened almond milk and a touch of honey can be a nutritious and indulgent-feeling snack.

Hydration should not be overlooked when it comes to smart snacking. Sometimes, what we perceive as hunger is actually thirst. Keeping a water bottle handy and sipping throughout the day can help prevent unnecessary snacking. Herbal teas or infused water can be a flavorful way to stay hydrated without adding calories.

Preparation is key to successful smart snacking. Having healthy options readily available can prevent reaching for less nutritious alternatives when hunger strikes. Spend some time each week preparing snacks like cut vegetables, portioned nuts, or homemade energy bars. Store these in clear containers at eye level in your fridge or pantry to make healthy choices the easy choice.

It's also important to be mindful of your snacking habits. Are you eating out of genuine hunger, or due to stress, boredom, or habit? Keeping a food diary for a week can help you identify patterns in your snacking behavior. If you find yourself snacking for reasons other than hunger, consider alternative activities like taking a short walk, practicing deep breathing, or engaging in a hobby.

For those leading particularly active lifestyles, snacks can play a crucial role in fueling workouts and supporting recovery. Pre-workout snacks should focus on easily digestible carbohydrates for quick energy, such as a banana or a small serving of oatmeal. Post-workout snacks should include a combination of carbohydrates and protein to replenish energy stores and support muscle recovery. A smoothie made with fruit, Greek yogurt, and a handful of spinach can be an excellent post-exercise option.

In conclusion, smart snacking is about making informed choices that support your overall health and nutritional goals. By focusing on nutrient-dense foods, practicing portion control, and being mindful of your snacking habits, you can turn snack time into an opportunity to nourish your body and maintain steady energy levels throughout the day. Remember, the goal is to find a balance that works for your lifestyle and preferences while supporting your long-term health.

Fruit-Based Desserts

Fruit-based desserts offer a delightful way to satisfy your sweet tooth while still maintaining a focus on health and nutrition. These desserts capitalize on the natural sweetness and vibrant flavors of fruits, often requiring little to no added sugars. By centering desserts around fruits, you can create treats that are not only delicious but also packed with vitamins, minerals, and fiber.

One of the primary advantages of fruit-based desserts is their versatility. Almost any fruit can be transformed into a delectable dessert with the right preparation. For example, baked apples stuffed with a mixture of oats, cinnamon, and a touch of honey can create a warm, comforting dessert that's reminiscent of apple pie but with a fraction of the calories and added sugars. Similarly, grilled peaches drizzled with a small amount of honey and topped with a dollop of Greek yogurt offer a simple yet elegant dessert that highlights the fruit's natural sweetness.

Berries are particularly well-suited for healthy desserts due to their high antioxidant content and natural sweetness. A mixed berry compote, gently simmered with a splash of balsamic vinegar, can be an excellent topping for Greek yogurt or used as a filling for crepes made with whole grain flour. For a more indulgent treat, dark chocolate-dipped strawberries provide antioxidants from both the fruit and the chocolate, while still feeling luxurious.

Frozen fruit desserts are another category that can satisfy cravings for something sweet and refreshing, especially during warmer months. Frozen banana "nice cream" has become increasingly popular as a healthier alternative to traditional ice cream. To make it, simply blend frozen banana chunks in a food processor until they reach a creamy consistency. This base can then be flavored with additions like cocoa powder, vanilla extract, or other frozen fruits to create a variety of flavors. Similarly, frozen grapes or cherries can serve as nature's candy, providing a sweet and refreshing snack with no preparation required.

For those who enjoy baking, incorporating fruits into baked goods can boost their nutritional value while adding moisture and flavor. Applesauce or mashed bananas can often be used to replace some or all of the oil in muffin or quick bread recipes, resulting in a lower-fat treat. Zucchini or carrots can be shredded and added to cakes or muffins, increasing the fiber and nutrient content while keeping the baked goods moist. When using fruits in baking, it's often possible to reduce the amount of added sugar in the recipe, as the fruits contribute their own natural sweetness.

Fruit-based pies and tarts can be made healthier by focusing on the fruit filling and minimizing the number of added sugars and fats. A whole grain or nut-based crust can add fiber and healthy fats, while a filling made primarily of fruit with just a small amount of sweetener can let the natural flavors shine. For a no-bake option, a fresh fruit tart with a date and nut crust, filled with Greek yogurt and topped with an array of sliced fruits, can be both visually appealing and nutritious.

Fruit leathers or roll-ups are another way to enjoy fruits in a dessert-like form. By pureeing fruits and spreading them thinly on a baking sheet to dehydrate in a low-temperature oven, you can create chewy, sweet treats without any added sugars. This method works well with a variety of fruits, from apples and pears to berries and tropical fruits like mangoes.

When creating fruit-based desserts, it's important to consider the ripeness and quality of the fruits you're using. Ripe, in-season fruits will have the best flavor and natural sweetness, often requiring little to no additional sweeteners. This not only makes for a healthier dessert but also supports sustainable eating practices by utilizing seasonal produce.

For those watching their sugar intake, even natural sugars from fruits should be consumed in moderation. While fruit-based desserts are generally healthier than their traditional counterparts, they still contain calories and sugars. The fiber in whole fruits helps to slow the absorption of these sugars, but it's still wise to be mindful of portion sizes.

Incorporating herbs and spices into fruit-based desserts can add complexity and interest without additional calories. A sprinkle of cinnamon or nutmeg can enhance the flavors of baked apples or pears, while a chiffonade of fresh mint can brighten a berry salad. Basil pairs surprisingly well with strawberries, and a touch of black pepper can intensify the flavor of fresh melon.

In conclusion, fruit-based desserts offer a wide array of options for satisfying your sweet cravings while maintaining a focus on health and nutrition. By leveraging the natural sweetness and flavors of fruits, and combining them with whole grains, nuts, and judicious use of sweeteners, you can create desserts that are not only delicious but also contribute positively to your overall diet. Whether you're enjoying a simple bowl of fresh berries or creating a more elaborate fruit-based tart, these desserts allow you to indulge your sweet tooth without compromising your health goals.

Healthier Baking Alternatives

Baking is often associated with indulgent treats high in sugar, refined flours, and unhealthy fats. However, with some creative substitutions and mindful ingredient choices, it's possible to transform traditional baked goods into healthier versions that still satisfy cravings. Healthier baking alternatives focus on increasing the nutritional value of baked goods while reducing less beneficial ingredients, resulting in treats that can be enjoyed as part of a balanced diet.

One of the primary strategies in healthier baking is to replace refined white flour with more nutritious alternatives. Whole wheat flour is a common substitute that adds fiber and nutrients, though it can result in a denser texture. For a lighter option, white whole wheat flour offers the nutritional benefits of whole grains with a milder flavor and lighter color. Almond flour, coconut flour, and oat flour are excellent gluten-free options that also add protein and healthy fats. When using these alternative flours, it's important to note that they often behave differently than all-purpose flour in recipes, sometimes requiring adjustments in liquid content or leavening agents.

Reducing sugar content is another key aspect of healthier baking. While sugar plays multiple roles in baking, including providing sweetness, contributing to texture, and aiding in browning, it's often possible to reduce the amount of sugar in a recipe by *25-30%* without significantly affecting the final product. Natural sweeteners like mashed bananas, applesauce, or dates can add sweetness while also contributing moisture and nutrients. Stevia, monk fruit extract, and erythritol are calorie-free sweeteners that can be used in baking, though they may require some experimentation to achieve the desired taste and texture.

Incorporating fruits and vegetables into baked goods is an excellent way to boost nutrition and add natural sweetness. Shredded zucchini or carrots can add moisture and nutrients to muffins or quick breads. Pureed pumpkin or sweet potato can replace some of the fat in recipes while adding flavor and vitamins. Unsweetened applesauce can often be substituted for some or all of the oil in a recipe, reducing fat content while maintaining moisture.

When it comes to fats, choosing healthier options can make a significant difference. Replacing saturated fats like butter with unsaturated fats like olive oil or avocado can improve the nutritional profile of baked goods. Greek yogurt or mashed avocado can often be used to replace some or all of the butter in a recipe, adding protein or healthy fats respectively. In some recipes, nut butters can serve as a flavorful fat replacement that also adds protein and fiber.

Eggs play a crucial role in many baked goods, providing structure, leavening, and moisture. For those looking to reduce cholesterol or follow a vegan diet, there are several egg alternatives that can be used in baking. Ground flaxseed or chia seeds mixed with water can create a gel-like substance that mimics the binding properties of eggs. Mashed bananas or commercial egg replacers can also be effective in many recipes.

Adding nuts, seeds, and dried fruits to baked goods can increase their nutritional value while adding texture and flavor. Chopped walnuts or almonds add healthy fats and protein, while chia seeds or ground flaxseed contribute omega-*3* fatty acids. When using dried fruits, look for varieties without added sugars to keep the overall sugar content in check.

For those with a chocolate craving, using high-quality dark chocolate (*70%* cocoa or higher) in place of milk chocolate can increase the antioxidant content while reducing sugar. Cocoa powder is another excellent way to add chocolate flavor without excessive calories or fat.

When it comes to leavening agents, using baking soda or baking powder in appropriate amounts is generally fine for healthy baking. However, for those watching their sodium intake, there are low-sodium baking powders available. In some recipes, the natural leavening power of ingredients like yogurt or buttermilk can be utilized to reduce the need for additional leavening agents.

It's worth noting that while these healthier baking alternatives can significantly improve the nutritional profile of baked goods, they should still be consumed in moderation as part of a balanced diet. Even healthier versions of cookies, cakes, and pastries are often calorie-dense and should be enjoyed mindfully.

Experimenting with healthier baking alternatives often requires some trial and error. Ingredients may behave differently than in traditional recipes, affecting texture, rise, and baking time. It's often helpful to start by making small substitutions and gradually increasing them as you become more comfortable with how different ingredients interact.

In conclusion, healthier baking alternatives offer a way to enjoy homemade treats while aligning with nutritional goals. By focusing on whole grain flours, reducing added sugars, incorporating fruits and vegetables, choosing healthier fats, and adding nutrient-dense ingredients like nuts and seeds, it's possible to create baked goods that are not only delicious but also contribute positively to overall health. With some creativity and willingness to experiment, you can transform your favorite baked treats into versions that satisfy both your taste buds and your nutritional needs.

Chapter 10: Cooking for Special Dietary Needs

In today's diverse culinary landscape, understanding and accommodating special dietary needs has become an essential skill for any health-conscious cook. Whether you're adapting your cooking for personal health reasons, catering to family members with specific dietary requirements, or simply expanding your culinary repertoire, this chapter will equip you with the knowledge and techniques to create delicious, nutritious meals that meet a variety of dietary needs. From gluten-free and dairy-free cooking to vegan, vegetarian, and low-sodium options, you'll discover how to navigate these dietary landscapes with confidence and creativity.

As we delve into the world of special diets, it's important to remember that these approaches to eating are not just trends, but often necessary lifestyle choices for many individuals. According to a study published in the Journal of the Academy of Nutrition and Dietetics, approximately *36%* of Americans follow a specific dietary pattern, with gluten-free, dairy-free, and plant-based diets among the most common[24]. By mastering the techniques and principles outlined in this chapter, you'll not only expand your culinary skills but also be better equipped to cater to a wider range of dietary needs, whether for yourself or others.

Throughout this chapter, we'll explore the fundamentals of each dietary approach, discussing the reasons behind these dietary choices, the key nutritional considerations, and the essential ingredients and cooking techniques that form the foundation of each style of eating. You'll learn how to adapt recipes, substitute ingredients, and create balanced meals that meet specific dietary requirements without compromising on flavor or nutrition. Moreover, we'll address the challenges often associated with special diets and provide practical solutions to ensure that your cooking remains diverse, enjoyable, and health-promoting.

As we navigate through gluten-free, dairy-free, vegan, vegetarian, and low-sodium cooking, keep in mind that these dietary approaches often overlap and can be combined to meet multiple dietary needs simultaneously. The skills you'll acquire in this chapter are transferable and will enhance your overall cooking repertoire, allowing you to create more inclusive meals that can be enjoyed by everyone at your table, regardless of their dietary restrictions.

Remember, cooking for special dietary needs is not about limitation, but rather about exploration and innovation. It's an opportunity to discover new ingredients, experiment with different cooking techniques, and develop a more nuanced understanding of flavor and nutrition. By the end of this chapter, you'll be well-equipped to tackle any dietary challenge with confidence, creativity, and culinary flair.

Gluten-Free Cooking Techniques

Gluten-free cooking has gained significant attention in recent years, not only for those with celiac disease or gluten sensitivity but also for individuals seeking to reduce their gluten intake for various health reasons. Gluten, a protein found in wheat, barley, and rye, can cause adverse reactions in some people, ranging from mild discomfort to severe autoimmune responses. Understanding the principles of gluten-free cooking is essential for creating safe, nutritious, and delicious meals for those following a gluten-free diet.

The first step in mastering gluten-free cooking is to familiarize yourself with gluten-free ingredients. Many naturally gluten-free foods form the foundation of a healthy diet, including fruits, vegetables, legumes, nuts, seeds, meat, poultry, fish, eggs, and dairy products. However, when it comes to grains and starches, you'll need to be more selective. Safe options include rice, quinoa, millet, amaranth, buckwheat, corn, and gluten-free oats. It's crucial to note that while these grains are naturally gluten-free, cross-contamination can occur during processing, so always look for certified gluten-free products when purchasing these items.

One of the biggest challenges in gluten-free cooking is replicating the texture and binding properties that gluten provides in traditional baking. Gluten gives structure to bread, pasta, and baked goods, making them elastic and chewy. To achieve similar results in gluten-free baking, you'll often need to use a combination of gluten-free flours and starches. Popular options include almond flour, coconut flour, rice flour, tapioca starch, potato starch, and xanthan gum. Each of these ingredients has unique properties and learning how to blend them effectively is key to successful gluten-free baking.

When adapting recipes to be gluten-free, it's important to understand that a simple one-to-one substitution of wheat flour with a gluten-free alternative often won't yield the desired results. Gluten-free flours absorb liquids differently and can affect the texture and structure of your dishes. As a general rule, start by replacing wheat flour with a gluten-free all-purpose flour blend, which typically contains a mix of gluten-free flours and starches. These blends are designed to mimic the properties of wheat flour and can be a good starting point for many recipes. However, be prepared to adjust the liquid content and baking times as needed.

In addition to baking, many savory dishes traditionally contain gluten, often in the form of thickeners or sauces. To create gluten-free versions of these dishes, you'll need to master alternative thickening techniques. Cornstarch, arrowroot powder, and potato starch are excellent gluten-free thickeners that can be used in place of wheat flour in gravies, sauces, and soups. When using these alternatives, remember that they have different thickening powers compared to wheat flour, so you may need to adjust the quantities used in your recipes.

Cross-contamination is a significant concern in gluten-free cooking, especially for those with celiac disease. Even tiny amounts of gluten can cause severe reactions in sensitive individuals. To prevent cross-contamination, it's essential to maintain a clean and organized kitchen. Use separate cutting boards, utensils, and cooking surfaces for gluten-free food preparation. If you're cooking both gluten-containing and gluten-free foods, always prepare the gluten-free items first and store them separately. Be particularly cautious with shared appliances like toasters and pasta makers, which can harbor gluten particles.

When it comes to flavor enhancement in gluten-free cooking, herbs, spices, and naturally gluten-free condiments become your best allies. Many commercial seasonings and sauces contain gluten, so it's important to either make your own or carefully read labels when purchasing. Experiment with fresh herbs, citrus zests, and gluten-free vinegars to add depth and complexity to your dishes. Remember that gluten-free doesn't mean flavor-free – with the right techniques and ingredients, your gluten-free meals can be just as delicious and satisfying as their gluten-containing counterparts.

Gluten-free cooking also presents an opportunity to explore a wider variety of grains and pseudocereals. Quinoa, for example, is not only gluten-free but also a complete protein, making it an excellent choice for those following a gluten-free diet. Buckwheat, despite its name, is not related to wheat and is naturally gluten-free. It has a nutty flavor and can be used in everything from pancakes to savory dishes. Experimenting with these diverse grains can add nutritional value and interesting textures to your meals.

As you become more comfortable with gluten-free cooking, you'll find that many traditional recipes can be easily adapted. For example, instead of using wheat-based pasta, try gluten-free alternatives made from rice, corn, or legumes. In place of wheat-based pizza crusts, experiment with cauliflower crusts or those made from gluten-free flours. The key is to approach gluten-free cooking with creativity and an open mind, seeing it as an opportunity to explore new flavors and textures rather than a limitation.

Lastly, it's important to remember that a gluten-free diet should still be a balanced one. Simply removing gluten from your diet doesn't automatically make it healthier. Focus on incorporating a variety of whole, nutrient-dense foods into your gluten-free meals. Include plenty of fruits, vegetables, lean proteins, and gluten-free whole grains to ensure you're meeting your nutritional needs. With practice and experimentation, you'll find that gluten-free cooking can be just as diverse, delicious, and satisfying as any other style of cooking.

Dairy-Free Alternatives

Dairy-free cooking has become increasingly popular, whether due to lactose intolerance, milk allergies, ethical considerations, or personal dietary preferences. The good news is that with the wide array of dairy alternatives available today, it's easier than ever to create delicious and nutritious dairy-free meals. This section will guide you through the world of dairy-free cooking, helping you understand how to substitute dairy products effectively while maintaining the flavor, texture, and nutritional balance of your favorite dishes.

The first step in mastering dairy-free cooking is to familiarize yourself with the various milk alternatives available. Plant-based milks such as almond, soy, oat, coconut, and rice milk can be used in place of cow's milk in most recipes. Each of these alternatives has its own unique flavor profile and nutritional composition. For example, soy milk is high in protein and works well in savory dishes, while almond milk has a slightly sweet, nutty flavor that's great for baking. Oat milk has gained popularity for its creamy texture, making it an excellent choice for coffee and tea. When choosing a milk alternative, consider both the flavor and the nutritional content, especially if you're relying on it as a significant source of nutrients like calcium and vitamin *D*.

Replacing cheese in dairy-free cooking can be more challenging, but there are numerous options available. Nutritional yeast, with its nutty, cheesy flavor, is a popular choice for adding a cheese-like taste to dishes. It's also a good source of *B* vitamins, including *B12*, which can be lacking in some plant-based diets. For texture, cashews can be soaked and blended to create a creamy base for sauces and dips. Commercial dairy-free cheeses, made from nuts, soy, or other plant-based ingredients, have also improved significantly in recent years and can be used in many recipes calling for traditional cheese.

When it comes to baking, replacing butter and cream can seem daunting, but there are many effective alternatives. Coconut oil can be used as a one-to-one replacement for butter in many recipes, providing a similar texture and richness. For a more neutral flavor, try using a high-quality vegetable oil or a dairy-free margarine. In recipes calling for cream, full-fat coconut milk can often be used as a substitute, particularly in curries and other savory dishes. For whipped cream, chilled coconut cream can be whipped to create a similar texture and mouthfeel.

Yogurt is another dairy product that's commonly used in cooking and baking. Fortunately, there are now many plant-based yogurt alternatives made from soy, coconut, almond, or oats. These can be used in place of dairy yogurt in most recipes, from breakfast parfaits to savory dips. When using these alternatives in baking, be aware that they may have a different moisture content than dairy yogurt, so you might need to adjust other liquids in the recipe accordingly.

One of the challenges of dairy-free cooking is ensuring that you're still getting adequate calcium and other nutrients typically found in dairy products. It's important to include other calcium-rich foods in your diet, such as leafy greens, fortified plant milks, tofu processed with calcium sulfate, and certain nuts and seeds. Many dairy-free alternatives are now fortified with calcium and vitamin *D* to help meet nutritional needs. However, if you're following a strict dairy-free diet, it's always a good idea to consult with a registered dietitian to ensure you're meeting all your nutritional requirements.

When adapting recipes to be dairy-free, it's often helpful to think about the function of the dairy product in the original recipe. Is it providing moisture, fat, protein, or flavor? Once you understand this, you can choose an appropriate substitute that fulfills the same role. For example, if a recipe calls for milk primarily for moisture, you might be able to use water or a plant-based milk. If it's for richness, a nut-based cream or coconut milk might be more appropriate.

Flavor is another important consideration in dairy-free cooking. Dairy products often add a rich, savory umami flavor to dishes. To replicate this in dairy-free cooking, you can use ingredients like miso paste, mushrooms, tomatoes, or seaweed, all of which are rich in umami compounds. These ingredients can add depth and complexity to your dishes, helping to create satisfying meals that don't leave you missing dairy.

It's worth noting that many cuisines around the world are naturally dairy-free or have dairy-free options. Asian cuisines, for example, often use coconut milk instead of dairy, while many African and Middle Eastern dishes rely on nuts and seeds for creaminess. Exploring these cuisines can provide inspiration and new techniques for your dairy-free cooking.

As with any dietary change, transitioning to dairy-free cooking may take some time and experimentation. Don't be discouraged if your first attempts don't turn out exactly as you hoped. With practice, you'll learn which substitutes work best in different recipes and how to adjust flavors and textures to your liking. Remember that dairy-free cooking isn't about perfectly replicating dairy-based dishes, but rather about creating delicious, satisfying meals that happen to be free from dairy.

Lastly, always read labels carefully when purchasing packaged foods, as dairy ingredients can be found in unexpected places. Look out for ingredients like whey, casein, and lactose, which are all derived from milk. With time, you'll become adept at identifying dairy-free products and ingredients, making your dairy-free cooking journey smoother and more enjoyable.

Vegan and Vegetarian Meal Ideas

Vegan and vegetarian diets have gained significant popularity in recent years, driven by a combination of health, environmental, and ethical considerations. Whether you're fully committed to a plant-based lifestyle or simply looking to incorporate more meatless meals into your diet, understanding the principles of vegan and vegetarian cooking can greatly expand your culinary repertoire. This section will explore a variety of delicious and nutritious meal ideas that cater to both vegan and vegetarian diets, demonstrating that plant-based eating can be both satisfying and diverse.

Before diving into specific meal ideas, it's important to understand the distinction between vegan and vegetarian diets. Vegetarians typically avoid meat, fish, and poultry, but may consume dairy products and eggs. Vegans, on the other hand, exclude all animal products, including dairy, eggs, and honey. Both diets can be nutritionally complete when well-planned, but it's crucial to ensure a balance of proteins, carbohydrates, healthy fats, vitamins, and minerals. Plant-based proteins such as legumes, nuts, seeds, and whole grains play a key role in these diets, as do a variety of fruits and vegetables to provide essential nutrients.

One of the cornerstones of successful vegan and vegetarian cooking is learning to create satisfying, protein-rich meals. Legumes, including beans, lentils, and chickpeas, are excellent sources of plant-based protein and can form the basis of many hearty dishes. For example, a classic three-bean chili made with kidney beans, black beans, and pinto beans, seasoned with cumin, chili powder, and smoked paprika, can be a warming and protein-packed meal. Serve it with brown rice or quinoa for a complete protein profile. Similarly, lentil-based dishes like dal, a staple in Indian cuisine, can be both nutritious and comforting. Try a red lentil dal spiced with turmeric, ginger, and garlic, served with whole grain naan or brown rice.

Tofu and tempeh, both derived from soybeans, are versatile ingredients that can be used in a variety of dishes. Firm tofu can be marinated and grilled for a meat-like texture, perfect for stir-fries or sandwiches. For example, a tofu banh mi sandwich with pickled vegetables and sriracha mayo (made with vegan mayonnaise) can be a delicious lunch option. Tempeh, with its nutty flavor and firm texture, works well in dishes like tempeh tacos or a tempeh bolognese sauce served over whole grain pasta.

Whole grains are another important component of vegan and vegetarian diets, providing both nutrients and satisfying textures. Grain bowls have become increasingly popular and are an excellent way to create balanced, customizable meals. Start with a base of quinoa, brown rice, or farro, then add a variety of roasted or raw vegetables, a plant-based protein source, and a flavorful dressing. For instance, a Mediterranean-inspired bowl might include quinoa, roasted eggplant and zucchini, chickpeas, cherry tomatoes, and a tahini-lemon dressing.

For those transitioning to a plant-based diet, it can be helpful to recreate familiar dishes using vegan or vegetarian ingredients. Cauliflower, for example, has proven to be an incredibly versatile ingredient. Roasted cauliflower steaks seasoned with herbs and spices can serve as a satisfying main course. Or, try a cauliflower-based alfredo sauce for a creamy pasta dish without the dairy. Simply blend steamed cauliflower with nutritional yeast, garlic, and plant-based milk for a rich, velvety sauce.

Nuts and seeds are not only great sources of protein and healthy fats but can also add texture and depth to plant-based dishes. A kale salad with roasted sweet potatoes, quinoa, pumpkin seeds, and a maple-mustard dressing can be a nutrient-dense meal that's both satisfying and delicious. For a heartier option, try stuffed bell peppers filled with a mixture of wild rice, lentils, walnuts, and herbs, baked until tender and topped with a cashew-based cream sauce.

Breakfast can sometimes be challenging for those new to vegan or vegetarian diets, but there are many delicious options beyond the standard cereal and plant milk. Overnight oats made with rolled oats, chia seeds, plant-based milk, and topped with fresh fruit and nuts can be a quick and nutritious start to the day. For a savory option, try a tofu scramble with turmeric, nutritional yeast, and your choice of vegetables, served with whole grain toast and avocado.

When it comes to baking, eggs and dairy are often key ingredients, but there are numerous plant-based alternatives that can yield delicious results. Aquafaba, the liquid from canned chickpeas, can be whipped to replace egg whites in many recipes. Flax or chia seeds mixed with water can act as a binder in place of eggs. For dairy, plant-based milks, coconut oil, and vegan butter can often be substituted one-to-one in recipes. Try making a vegan banana bread using mashed bananas, almond milk, and coconut oil for a moist, flavorful treat.

It's important to remember that vegan and vegetarian cooking is not about deprivation, but rather about exploring the vast world of plant-based ingredients. Experimenting with different cuisines can open up a world of naturally vegan or vegetarian dishes. Indian cuisine, for example, offers a wealth of vegetarian options, from spicy vegetable curries to crispy dosas filled with spiced potatoes. Middle Eastern cuisine is another great source of inspiration, with dishes like falafel, hummus, and tabbouleh (Tabouli) that are naturally vegan and packed with flavor.

Lastly, don't forget about the importance of umami flavors in creating satisfying plant-based meals. Ingredients like mushrooms, tomatoes, miso paste, and nutritional yeast can add depth and savory notes to your dishes. A mushroom risotto made with arborio rice, a variety of mushrooms, and finished with nutritional yeast can be a comforting and luxurious meal that doesn't leave you missing meat or dairy.

As you explore vegan and vegetarian cooking, remember that balance is key. Aim to include a variety of fruits, vegetables, whole grains, legumes, nuts, and seeds in your diet to ensure you're getting a full range of nutrients. With creativity and an open mind, you'll find that plant-based cooking can be an exciting culinary adventure, offering endless possibilities for delicious, nutritious meals.

Low-Sodium Cooking Strategies

Reducing sodium intake is a common dietary goal for many individuals, particularly those managing hypertension, heart disease, or kidney problems. However, creating flavorful low-sodium meals can be challenging, as salt is often relied upon as a primary flavor enhancer in cooking. This section will explore strategies for low-sodium cooking that don't compromise on taste, helping you create delicious meals while keeping your sodium intake in check.

The first step in low-sodium cooking is understanding where sodium comes from in our diets. While table salt is an obvious source, many processed and packaged foods contain high levels of hidden sodium. Canned soups, deli meats, cheese, and even bread can be significant contributors to daily sodium intake. By focusing on whole, unprocessed foods and cooking from scratch, you can have much greater control over the sodium content of your meals.

One of the most effective strategies for low-sodium cooking is to enhance flavors using herbs and spices. Fresh herbs like basil, cilantro, parsley, and mint can add bright, fresh flavors to dishes without the need for salt. Dried herbs and spices such as oregano, thyme, cumin, paprika, and chili powder can provide depth and complexity to your cooking. Experiment with different combinations to find flavor profiles you enjoy. For example, a Mediterranean-inspired blend of oregano, basil, and garlic can transform a simple chicken dish, while a mix of cumin, coriander, and turmeric can give vegetables a warm, earthy flavor.

Acidic ingredients are another powerful tool in low-sodium cooking. Lemon juice, lime juice, vinegars, and wine can all add brightness and depth to dishes, helping to compensate for reduced salt. A splash of balsamic vinegar can elevate a simple tomato sauce, while a squeeze of lemon juice can brighten up a fish dish or a vegetable stir-fry. Citrus zest is another great way to add intense flavor without sodium – try adding lemon or orange zest to marinades or dressings for an extra flavor boost.

Umami-rich ingredients can also help create satisfying flavors in low-sodium cooking. Mushrooms, tomatoes, aged cheeses (used sparingly), and fermented foods like miso paste (look for low-sodium varieties) can all contribute savory, complex flavors to dishes. Roasting or grilling vegetables can intensify their natural flavors and add a depth that might otherwise be achieved with salt. For example, a pasta sauce made with slow-roasted tomatoes and garlic can be incredibly flavorful without the need for added salt.

When it comes to seasoning meats and fish, consider using dry rubs made from a blend of herbs and spices instead of salt-based marinades. A mixture of paprika, garlic powder, onion powder, and black pepper can create a flavorful crust on grilled chicken or fish. For red meat, a rub of ground coffee, cocoa powder, and chili can add rich, complex flavors without relying on salt.

In baking, where salt often plays a crucial role in flavor and texture, reducing sodium can be more challenging. However, there are strategies you can employ. In bread recipes, you can often reduce the salt by up to 50% without significantly affecting the rise or texture. In sweet baked goods, try enhancing flavors with vanilla extract, almond extract, or citrus zest to compensate for reduced salt. When a recipe calls for salted butter, use unsalted and adjust the seasoning yourself, allowing for greater control over the sodium content.

Cooking techniques can also play a role in enhancing flavor without salt. Browning meats and vegetables thoroughly can develop rich, complex flavors through the Maillard reaction. Slow cooking can allow flavors to develop and meld over time, creating depth without the need for excessive seasoning. For example, a low-sodium vegetable soup can become incredibly flavorful when simmered slowly, allowing the natural flavors of the ingredients to intensify.

When using canned goods, which are often high in sodium, look for low-sodium or no-salt-added varieties. Alternatively, you can rinse canned beans and vegetables thoroughly to remove excess sodium.

Better yet, cook dried beans from scratch, which allows you complete control over seasoning. A pot of beans cooked with aromatics like onion, garlic, and bay leaves can be incredibly flavorful without any added salt.

Creating your own spice blends and seasoning mixes is another effective strategy for low-sodium cooking. Commercial seasoning blends often contain high levels of salt, but by making your own, you can create flavorful combinations without the added sodium. A simple Italian seasoning blend of dried basil, oregano, rosemary, and thyme can be used to flavor everything from roasted vegetables to homemade tomato sauce.

It's important to note that as you reduce sodium in your cooking, your palate will gradually adjust. Foods that initially taste bland will begin to taste properly seasoned as your taste buds become more sensitive to subtle flavors. This adjustment period can take a few weeks, so be patient with yourself as you adapt to a lower-sodium diet.

Lastly, remember that low-sodium cooking doesn't mean no-sodium cooking. Small amounts of salt used strategically can still have a big impact on flavor. When you do use salt, opt for sea salt or kosher salt, which have a purer flavor than table salt and may allow you to use less overall. Adding a small pinch of salt at the end of cooking can often provide a satisfying flavor boost without significantly increasing the overall sodium content of the dish.

By incorporating these strategies into your cooking routine, you can create delicious, flavorful meals while keeping your sodium intake in check. Low-sodium cooking is an opportunity to explore new flavors and techniques, ultimately leading to a more diverse and exciting culinary experience.

Chapter 11: Enhancing Flavor Naturally

In the journey of mastering healthy cooking, one of the most crucial skills to develop is the ability to enhance flavors naturally. This chapter delves into the art and science of creating delicious, satisfying meals without relying on excessive salt, sugar, or unhealthy fats. By harnessing the power of herbs, spices, and other natural flavor enhancers, you can transform simple, wholesome ingredients into culinary masterpieces that nourish both body and soul.

The importance of flavor in healthy cooking cannot be overstated. When food tastes good, you're more likely to enjoy it, feel satisfied, and stick to your healthy eating goals. Moreover, many natural flavor enhancers come with their own set of health benefits, from antioxidants in herbs to anti-inflammatory compounds in spices. By learning to use these ingredients effectively, you'll not only create more appetizing dishes but also boost the nutritional value of your meals.

Throughout this chapter, you'll discover a wide array of techniques and ingredients that can elevate your cooking. From the subtle aromatics of fresh herbs to the bold punch of spice blends, from tangy marinades to umami-rich sauces, you'll explore a world of flavors that can make healthy eating a truly enjoyable experience. You'll learn how to balance flavors, create depth in your dishes, and adapt these techniques to suit your personal taste preferences and dietary needs.

As you progress through the sections, keep in mind that flavor enhancement is both an art and a science. While there are general principles to follow, don't be afraid to experiment and trust your palate. The more you practice and explore, the more intuitive your cooking will become. Remember, the goal is not just to make food that's good for you, but to create dishes that you genuinely look forward to eating.

So, let's embark on this flavorful journey and discover how to make healthy cooking not just nutritious, but truly delicious. By the end of this chapter, you'll have a robust toolkit of flavor-enhancing techniques that will revolutionize your approach to healthy cooking and eating.

Cooking with Herbs and Spices

Herbs and spices are the cornerstone of flavor enhancement in healthy cooking. These powerhouse ingredients not only add depth, aroma, and complexity to your dishes but also come packed with health benefits. From boosting metabolism to reducing inflammation, herbs and spices are nature's way of making food both delicious and nutritious. In this section, we'll explore how to select, store, and use a variety of herbs and spices to elevate your cooking.

Let's start with fresh herbs. These leafy greens can transform a dish with their bright, vibrant flavors. Basil, cilantro, parsley, mint, and dill are just a few examples of herbs that can add a fresh, lively note to your meals. When using fresh herbs, it's generally best to add them towards the end of cooking to preserve their delicate flavors. For example, toss chopped basil into your pasta just before serving, or sprinkle fresh cilantro over a bowl of chili as a finishing touch. To store fresh herbs, wrap them loosely in a damp paper towel and place them in a plastic bag in the refrigerator. Most will last about a week when stored properly.

Dried herbs, on the other hand, have a more concentrated flavor and can withstand longer cooking times. They're excellent for use in slow-cooked dishes, marinades, and spice rubs. When substituting dried herbs for fresh in a recipe, use about one-third of the amount called for, as dried herbs are more potent. Some versatile dried herbs to keep in your pantry include oregano, thyme, rosemary, and sage. Store dried herbs in airtight containers away from heat and light to preserve their flavor.

Spices open up a world of flavors from cultures around the globe. From the warmth of cinnamon and nutmeg to the heat of cayenne and black pepper, spices can add complexity and depth to your dishes. Experiment with spice blends like curry powder, za'atar, or garam masala to easily add authentic flavors to your cooking. When using spices, remember that a little can go a long way. Start with small amounts and adjust to taste. To bring out the full flavor of spices, try toasting them in a dry pan over medium heat until fragrant before adding them to your dish.

One effective way to incorporate herbs and spices into your cooking is through creating your own spice blends. This allows you to customize flavors to your liking and avoid the additives often found in store-bought mixes. A simple Italian herb blend might include dried basil, oregano, thyme, and rosemary. For a Moroccan-inspired mix, combine cumin, coriander, cinnamon, and paprika. These homemade blends can be stored in airtight containers and used to quickly add flavor to everything from roasted vegetables to grilled meats.

It's important to note that herbs and spices do more than just add flavor; many have significant health benefits. For instance, turmeric, a bright yellow spice common in Indian cuisine, contains curcumin, a compound with powerful anti-inflammatory properties[25]. Cinnamon has been shown to help regulate blood sugar levels, making it a great addition to breakfast dishes or baked goods[26].

By incorporating a variety of herbs and spices into your cooking, you're not just enhancing flavor, but also boosting the nutritional value of your meals.

When it comes to pairing herbs and spices with different foods, there are some classic combinations to keep in mind. Rosemary and thyme pair beautifully with roasted meats and root vegetables. Basil is a natural companion to tomatoes and other Mediterranean flavors. Cumin and coriander are essential in many Mexican and Indian dishes. However, don't be afraid to experiment and create your own unique flavor combinations. The key is to start with small amounts and taste as you go, adjusting the flavors to suit your palate.

Remember, the goal of using herbs and spices in healthy cooking is not to mask the natural flavors of whole foods, but to enhance and complement them. Use these flavor boosters to bring out the best in fresh vegetables, lean proteins, and whole grains. With practice, you'll develop an intuitive sense of how to use herbs and spices to create delicious, satisfying meals that support your health goals.

Healthy Marinades and Rubs

Marinades and rubs are powerful tools in the healthy cook's arsenal, capable of infusing foods with intense flavors while often reducing the need for added fats or excessive salt. These techniques are particularly useful for enhancing lean proteins and vegetables, turning simple ingredients into flavorful, satisfying meals. In this section, we'll explore how to create and use healthy marinades and rubs to elevate your cooking.

Let's start with marinades. A marinade is a liquid mixture that foods, particularly meats and vegetables, are soaked in before cooking. The purpose of a marinade is twofold: to add flavor and, in some cases, to tenderize. A basic marinade typically consists of an acid (like citrus juice or vinegar), oil, and flavorings (such as herbs, spices, and aromatics). The acid helps break down tough fibers in meat, making it more tender, while also penetrating the food with flavor. However, it's important to note that marinating doesn't necessarily make meat more moist; that's more a function of cooking technique.

When creating healthy marinades, focus on using ingredients that pack a flavor punch without adding unnecessary calories or unhealthy fats. Citrus juices, vinegars, and low-sodium soy sauce or tamari make excellent bases for marinades. These acidic ingredients not only add flavor but also help tenderize meats. For oil, opt for heart-healthy options like olive oil or avocado oil, but use them sparingly. Many traditional marinade recipes call for more oil than is necessary; you can often reduce the amount by half or more without sacrificing flavor.

Here's a simple formula for creating a healthy marinade: combine *1*-part acid (like lemon juice or vinegar), *1*-part oil, and *1*-part flavorings (like minced garlic, herbs, and spices). For example, a Mediterranean-inspired marinade might include lemon juice, olive oil, minced garlic, dried oregano, and black pepper. An Asian-inspired marinade could combine rice vinegar, a small amount of sesame oil, grated ginger, low-sodium soy sauce, and a touch of honey for balance.

When marinating, always do so in the refrigerator to prevent bacterial growth. The length of marinating time depends on the food. Delicate proteins like fish or tofu only need *30* minutes to an hour, while tougher cuts of meat can marinate for several hours or overnight. Vegetables can generally marinate for *30* minutes to *2* hours. Avoid marinating for too long, especially with acidic marinades, as this can actually toughen the meat or break down vegetables too much.

Now, let's turn our attention to rubs. A rub is a mixture of dry ingredients that is applied directly to the surface of food before cooking. Rubs are an excellent way to add flavor without adding moisture, making them perfect for cooking methods like grilling or roasting where you want to achieve a crispy exterior. Rubs can be applied just before cooking or left on for several hours to allow the flavors to penetrate the food.

Creating a healthy rub is all about balancing flavors without relying too heavily on salt. Start with a base of herbs and spices, then add a small amount of salt if desired. For example, a basic *BBQ* rub might include paprika, garlic powder, onion powder, black pepper, and a touch of brown sugar for balance.

A Mexican-inspired rub could combine chili powder, cumin, oregano, and a small amount of salt. Remember, you can always add more salt at the table if needed, but starting with less in your cooking allows you to better control your sodium intake.

When applying a rub, start by patting the food dry with paper towels. This helps the rub adhere better and promotes better browning during cooking. Apply the rub generously, pressing it into the surface of the food. For the best flavor, apply the rub at least *30* minutes before cooking to allow the flavors to penetrate. For even more flavor, you can apply the rub the night before and let the food sit in the refrigerator overnight.

Both marinades and rubs offer opportunities to experiment with global flavors. A Jamaican jerk rub might include allspice, thyme, and scotch bonnet pepper. A Middle Eastern marinade could feature lemon juice, olive oil, garlic, and za'atar spice blend. By exploring different flavor profiles, you can keep your healthy meals exciting and varied.

It's worth noting that marinades and rubs aren't just for meat. They can be excellent ways to add flavor to plant-based proteins like tofu, tempeh, or seitan. They're also great for vegetables, whether you're grilling, roasting, or even preparing raw veggies for a salad. A simple herb rub can transform plain roasted vegetables, while a tangy marinade can make a delicious base for a vegetable stir-fry.

Remember, the key to using marinades and rubs in healthy cooking is to focus on flavor-packed ingredients rather than relying on excessive salt or sugar. With these techniques in your culinary toolkit, you'll be able to create delicious, satisfying meals that support your health goals while tantalizing your taste buds.

Nutritious Dressings and Sauces

Dressings and sauces are the unsung heroes of healthy cooking. They have the power to transform simple, wholesome ingredients into exciting, flavorful meals. However, many store-bought versions are laden with unhealthy fats, added sugars, and excessive sodium. By learning to make your own nutritious dressings and sauces, you can control the ingredients while creating flavors tailored to your preferences. In this section, we'll explore how to craft delicious, health-promoting dressings and sauces that will elevate your meals.

Let's start with salad dressings, as they're often the first thing people think of when it comes to sauces in healthy cooking. A basic vinaigrette is a great place to begin. The classic ratio is *3* parts oil to 1 part vinegar, but for a lighter dressing, you can shift this to *2:1* or even *1:1*. Choose heart-healthy oils like extra virgin olive oil, avocado oil, or walnut oil. For the acid, experiment with different vinegars (balsamic, apple cider, red wine) or citrus juices. Add herbs, spices, or a touch of mustard for extra flavor. For example, a simple lemon-herb vinaigrette might include lemon juice, olive oil, minced garlic, dried oregano, and a touch of Dijon mustard.

Creamy dressings don't have to be off-limits in healthy cooking. Instead of using mayonnaise or sour cream as a base, try Greek yogurt, mashed avocado, or pureed soft tofu. These alternatives provide creaminess along with beneficial nutrients. A healthy ranch dressing could be made with Greek yogurt, lemon juice, garlic powder, onion powder, and fresh herbs like dill and chives. For a vegan option, blend soaked cashews with water, lemon juice, and seasonings to create a creamy base.

When it comes to sauces, the possibilities are endless. A simple tomato sauce can be made by sautéing garlic and onions in a small amount of olive oil, then adding canned crushed tomatoes, herbs like basil and oregano, and simmering until thickened. This homemade version allows you to control the sodium and avoid added sugars often found in jarred sauces. For a creamier sauce without the cream, try pureeing roasted red peppers with garlic, olive oil, and a touch of vegetable broth. This makes a delicious, nutrient-rich sauce for pasta or grilled vegetables.

Pesto is another versatile sauce that can be made healthier. Traditional pesto is high in calories due to large amounts of oil and cheese. Try reducing the oil and replacing some of the cheese with nutritional yeast for a lighter version. You can also experiment with different greens beyond basil - spinach, kale, or arugula can make delicious and nutrient-dense pestos. For example, a kale and walnut pesto might include kale leaves, walnuts, garlic, lemon juice, a small amount of Parmesan, and olive oil, all blended until smooth.

Asian-inspired sauces can add a burst of flavor to stir-fries and grain bowls. A basic stir-fry sauce might include low-sodium soy sauce or tamari, rice vinegar, a small amount of sesame oil, grated ginger, and garlic. For sweetness, use a small amount of honey or maple syrup instead of sugar. Thicken the sauce with a slurry of cornstarch and water instead of using store-bought sauces that often contain added sugars and preservatives.

When creating sauces, consider incorporating ingredients that not only add flavor but also boost nutritional value. For instance, adding pureed vegetables to sauces can increase fiber and nutrient content. A cauliflower Alfredo sauce, made by blending steamed cauliflower with garlic, a small amount of Parmesan, and vegetable broth, is a great low-calorie alternative to traditional cream-based Alfredo.

Herbs can be the basis for flavorful, nutrient-rich sauces. Chimichurri, a sauce originating from Argentina, is made with parsley, garlic, olive oil, and vinegar. It's packed with flavor and antioxidants, making it a healthy choice to drizzle over grilled meats or vegetables. Similarly, an Italian salsa verde, made with parsley, capers, anchovies, and olive oil, can add a burst of flavor to fish or chicken dishes.

Remember, a little sauce can go a long way in terms of flavor. Instead of drowning your food in sauce, try using it as a flavor accent. This approach not only keeps calories in check but also allows the natural flavors of your ingredients to shine through. When storing homemade dressings and sauces, keep them in airtight containers in the refrigerator. Most will last for about a week, allowing you to prep ahead for quick and flavorful meals throughout the week.

By mastering the art of making nutritious dressings and sauces, you'll have a powerful tool for making healthy meals more appealing and satisfying. These homemade versions allow you to control the ingredients, reduce unnecessary additives, and tailor flavors to your liking. With practice, you'll find that creating delicious, healthy sauces becomes second nature, opening up a world of culinary possibilities in your health-conscious kitchen.

Incorporating Umami Flavors

Umami, often described as the fifth taste alongside sweet, sour, salty, and bitter, is a savory, meaty flavor that can add depth and satisfaction to your dishes. Understanding and incorporating umami flavors is a powerful technique in healthy cooking, as it can make plant-based and low-fat dishes taste richer and more satisfying without adding excessive calories or unhealthy ingredients. In this section, we'll explore the science of umami and how to harness its flavor-enhancing properties in your journey to healthy cooking.

Umami was first identified by Japanese chemist Kikunae Ikeda in *1908*, who isolated glutamates as the source of the savory taste in kombu seaweed. Scientifically, umami is the taste of glutamates and nucleotides, which are present in many foods. These compounds stimulate specific receptors on our tongues, creating the characteristic savory flavor we associate with umami. Interestingly, the presence of umami flavors can also enhance our perception of other tastes, making food seem more flavorful overall[27].

One of the most common sources of umami in Western cuisine is tomatoes, particularly when they're cooked or concentrated. This is why tomato paste can be such a powerful flavor enhancer in sauces and stews. Other vegetable sources of umami include mushrooms (especially dried mushrooms), fermented products like soy sauce and miso, and aged cheeses like Parmesan. In the realm of proteins, meats (particularly when browned), fish, and seafood are rich in umami compounds.

Incorporating umami flavors into your healthy cooking can be as simple as adding a small amount of Parmesan cheese to a vegetable dish or using mushrooms in a plant-based burger. However, to truly harness the power of umami, consider these techniques:

- Use tomato paste: A tablespoon of tomato paste can add depth to soups, stews, and sauces without adding significant calories. Try sautéing it briefly in oil before adding other ingredients to enhance its flavor.
- Incorporate dried mushrooms: Rehydrate dried mushrooms and use both the mushrooms and their soaking liquid to add umami depth to dishes. Dried shiitake mushrooms are particularly rich in umami compounds.
- Experiment with fermented products: Small amounts of miso paste, soy sauce, or nutritional yeast can add a savory boost to many dishes. Be mindful of sodium content when using soy sauce or miso.
- Roast vegetables: Roasting intensifies the natural umami in vegetables like tomatoes, mushrooms, and bell peppers. Use these as a base for sauces or as toppings for grain bowls.
- Try seaweed: Kombu, nori, and other seaweeds are rich in glutamates. Use them in broths or as seasoning for rice dishes.

One powerful umami-boosting technique is to create a vegetable-based broth or stock. Start by roasting a mix of umami-rich vegetables like mushrooms, tomatoes, and garlic. Then simmer these with aromatics like onions and celery, along with herbs and a small piece of kombu seaweed. The resulting broth will be packed with umami flavor and can be used as a base for soups, sauces, or for cooking grains.

Another strategy is to create umami-rich condiments that can be added to dishes as needed. For example, a mushroom-based "flavor bomb" can be made by finely chopping mushrooms and slowly cooking them down with a bit of soy sauce and balsamic vinegar until they form a paste. This concentrated umami paste can be stirred into soups, spread on sandwiches, or used as a marinade for proteins.

When incorporating umami flavors, it's important to balance them with other tastes. Umami pairs particularly well with acidic flavors, which is why tomatoes (which are both umami-rich and acidic) are so versatile. Try balancing umami-rich ingredients with a splash of vinegar or citrus juice to create a more complex flavor profile.

It's worth noting that while many umami-rich ingredients are healthy in moderation, some (like aged cheeses and cured meats) should be used sparingly in a health-conscious diet due to their high sodium or saturated fat content. Focus on plant-based sources of umami when possible, and use animal-based sources as flavor accents rather than main ingredients.

By understanding and incorporating umami flavors, you can create satisfying, flavorful meals that support your health goals. Whether you're trying to reduce meat consumption, cut back on added fats, or simply make vegetables more appealing, umami can be a powerful ally in your healthy cooking toolkit. With practice, you'll develop an intuitive sense of how to use umami-rich ingredients to enhance the flavor and satisfaction of your meals, making healthy eating a truly enjoyable experience.

Chapter 12: Practicing Mindful Eating

In the journey towards a healthier lifestyle, the focus often falls on what we eat, but equally important is how we eat. Mindful eating is a powerful practice that can transform your relationship with food, enhance your enjoyment of meals, and contribute significantly to your overall well-being. This chapter delves into the art of mindful eating, exploring techniques to bring awareness to your eating habits, understand portion control, address emotional eating, and ultimately find joy in the nourishing foods you prepare.

Mindful eating is rooted in the broader concept of mindfulness, which involves being fully present and engaged in the current moment. When applied to eating, this practice encourages you to pay attention to the sensory experience of your food, your body's hunger and fullness cues, and the thoughts and emotions that arise during meals. By cultivating this awareness, you can develop a more balanced and positive approach to nutrition that goes beyond calorie counting or restrictive diets.

Throughout this chapter, you'll discover practical strategies to incorporate mindfulness into your meals, learn how to recognize and respond to your body's true hunger signals, and explore ways to make eating a more intentional and satisfying experience. Whether you're looking to improve your digestion, manage your weight, or simply enjoy your food more deeply, the principles of mindful eating can be a valuable addition to your healthy cooking journey.

Mindfulness Techniques for Eating

Mindful eating begins with bringing your full attention to the act of eating. This means slowing down, engaging all your senses, and creating an environment conducive to awareness. One fundamental technique is to practice eating without distractions. Turn off the television, put away your phone, and step away from your computer. By eliminating these distractions, you create space to focus solely on your meal and the experience of eating.

Another key technique is to eat slowly and chew thoroughly. Take smaller bites and chew each mouthful *20* to *30* times before swallowing. This not only aids in digestion but also allows you to fully taste and appreciate your food. As you chew, pay attention to the flavors, textures, and aromas of your meal. Notice how these sensations change as you continue to chew. This practice can enhance your enjoyment of food and help you feel more satisfied with smaller portions.

Engaging all your senses is a powerful mindfulness technique. Before you begin eating, take a moment to observe your food. Notice the colors, shapes, and arrangement on your plate. Inhale deeply and savor the aroma. As you take your first bite, focus on the temperature and texture in your mouth. Listen to the sounds of your chewing. By fully engaging your senses, you create a richer, more satisfying eating experience.

Practicing gratitude is another important aspect of mindful eating. Before your meal, take a moment to reflect on the journey your food has taken to reach your plate. Consider the farmers who grew the ingredients, the workers who transported them, and the effort you put into preparing the meal. This practice can foster a deeper appreciation for your food and a sense of connection to the broader food system.

Mindful eating also involves checking in with your body throughout the meal. Pause periodically to assess your level of fullness. Use a hunger-fullness scale, where *1* is extremely hungry and *10* is uncomfortably full. Aim to start eating when you're at *3* or *4* (slightly hungry) and stop when you reach *7* or *8* (comfortably full but not stuffed). This practice helps you tune into your body's natural hunger and fullness cues, preventing overeating.

Another technique to enhance mindfulness during meals is to use chopsticks or smaller utensils. This naturally slows down your eating pace and encourages you to take smaller bites. If you're not accustomed to using chopsticks, the extra concentration required can help keep your mind focused on the act of eating.

Incorporating mindful breathing into your meals can also be beneficial. Before you begin eating, take a few deep breaths to center yourself. Throughout the meal, pause occasionally to take a deep breath. This can help you stay present and relaxed, enhancing your ability to tune into your body's signals.

Lastly, consider keeping a mindful eating journal. After each meal, jot down what you ate, how you felt before and after eating, and any observations about your eating experience. This practice can help you identify patterns in your eating habits and increase your overall awareness of your relationship with food.

By consistently practicing these mindfulness techniques, you can transform your meals from routine activities into opportunities for nourishment, enjoyment, and self-awareness. Over time, these practices can lead to a more balanced and intuitive approach to eating that supports your overall health and well-being.

Understanding Portion Control

Portion control is a crucial aspect of mindful eating and plays a significant role in maintaining a healthy diet. In a world where oversized portions have become the norm, understanding and implementing proper portion sizes can be challenging. However, mastering this skill is essential for managing calorie intake, maintaining a healthy weight, and ensuring balanced nutrition.

The first step in understanding portion control is recognizing that portion sizes have grown significantly over the past few decades. A study published in the American Journal of Public Health found that portion sizes for many common foods have increased by *2* to *5* times since the *1970s*[28]. This "portion distortion" has led many people to overeat without realizing it. By becoming aware of appropriate portion sizes, you can take control of your food intake and make more informed choices.

One effective strategy for portion control is to use visual cues to estimate serving sizes. For example, a serving of meat should be about the size of a deck of cards or the palm of your hand. A serving of grains or pasta should be about the size of your fist. For vegetables, aim for a serving size that would fit in two cupped hands. These visual references can be particularly helpful when eating out or in situations where you can't measure your food precisely.

Another useful tool for portion control is to use smaller plates and bowls. Research has shown that the size of your dinnerware can significantly influence how much you eat. A study published in the Journal of Consumer Research found that people served themselves 31% more ice cream when using a large bowl compared to a smaller one[29]. By using smaller plates, you can create the illusion of a full plate with less food, helping you feel satisfied with smaller portions.

When it comes to packaged foods, don't assume that the entire package is a single serving. Always check the nutrition label to see how many servings are in the container. If possible, portion out single servings into separate containers or bags. This can prevent mindless overeating, especially with snack foods.

For home-cooked meals, consider measuring your ingredients and using recipes that provide clear serving sizes. This can help you become more familiar with appropriate portion sizes and make it easier to replicate balanced meals. Over time, you'll develop a better intuitive sense of proper portions without needing to measure everything.

It's also important to understand the concept of energy density when considering portion sizes. Foods with high energy density contain more calories per gram, while those with low energy density have fewer calories for the same volume. Vegetables, fruits, and broth-based soups are examples of low energy-dense foods that allow you to eat larger portions for fewer calories. On the other hand, foods like nuts, cheese, and oils are energy-dense and should be consumed in smaller portions.

When dining out, where portion sizes are often much larger than necessary, consider strategies like sharing a meal with a dining companion, ordering an appetizer as your main course, or immediately boxing up half of your meal to take home. These approaches can help you enjoy restaurant meals without overindulging.

Remember that portion control doesn't mean depriving yourself or never enjoying your favorite foods. Instead, it's about finding a balance that allows you to nourish your body appropriately while still enjoying your meals. By combining portion control with mindful eating techniques, you can create a sustainable approach to healthy eating that doesn't feel restrictive.

Lastly, be patient with yourself as you learn to implement portion control. It takes time to adjust to appropriate serving sizes, especially if you're used to larger portions. Start by making small changes and gradually work towards more balanced portions. With practice and consistency, proper portion control will become second nature, supporting your overall health and nutrition goals.

Addressing Emotional Eating

Emotional eating is a common challenge that many people face on their journey to healthier eating habits. It refers to the tendency to use food to cope with emotions, rather than to satisfy physical hunger. Understanding and addressing emotional eating is crucial for developing a balanced relationship with food and maintaining overall well-being.

The first step in addressing emotional eating is to recognize its signs. Emotional hunger often comes on suddenly, craves specific comfort foods, and isn't satisfied even after you're full. It's often accompanied by mindless eating and feelings of guilt afterward. In contrast, physical hunger develops gradually, is open to various food options, and stops when you're full. By learning to distinguish between emotional and physical hunger, you can begin to make more conscious choices about when and why you eat.

Identifying your emotional eating triggers is another important step. Common triggers include stress, boredom, loneliness, anxiety, and even positive emotions like happiness or excitement. Keep a food and mood journal for a few weeks, noting what you eat, when you eat, how you feel before and after eating, and your hunger level. This can help you spot patterns and identify specific emotions or situations that lead to emotional eating.

Once you've identified your triggers, work on developing alternative coping strategies. If stress is a major trigger, consider stress-reduction techniques like deep breathing, meditation, or yoga. For boredom, create a list of engaging activities you can turn to instead of food, such as reading, calling a friend, or pursuing a hobby. If loneliness triggers emotional eating, focus on building meaningful connections and social support.

Practicing mindfulness can be particularly effective in addressing emotional eating. When you feel the urge to eat, pause and check in with yourself. Ask yourself if you're truly hungry or if you're seeking food for emotional reasons. If it's the latter, try to sit with the emotion for a few minutes without immediately reaching for food. This can help you develop greater emotional awareness and resilience.

It's also important to ensure you're meeting your basic needs. Sometimes, what seems like emotional hunger is actually a sign that you're not getting enough sleep, hydration, or balanced nutrition. Prioritize regular, balanced meals and adequate sleep to help stabilize your mood and energy levels, which can reduce the likelihood of emotional eating.

When you do find yourself eating for emotional reasons, approach the situation with compassion rather than judgment. Emotional eating is a learned coping mechanism, and it takes time to develop new habits. Instead of berating yourself, use the experience as an opportunity to learn and grow. Reflect on what led to the emotional eating episode and how you might handle similar situations differently in the future.

Consider seeking support if emotional eating is a significant struggle for you. This could involve talking to a trusted friend or family member, joining a support group, or working with a therapist or registered dietitian who specializes in emotional eating. Professional support can provide valuable tools and strategies for addressing the root causes of emotional eating and developing healthier coping mechanisms.

It's also worth examining your overall relationship with food. Restrictive diets or labeling foods as "good" or "bad" can actually increase the likelihood of emotional eating. Instead, work on developing a balanced, flexible approach to eating that allows for occasional indulgences without guilt. This can help reduce the allure of "forbidden" foods and make it easier to eat mindfully.

Finally, remember that food does have an emotional component, and that's not inherently bad. Food is often tied to cultural traditions, celebrations, and social connections. The goal is not to eliminate all emotional connections to food, but rather to ensure that emotions aren't the primary driver of your eating habits. By developing a more balanced relationship with food, you can enjoy its emotional and social aspects while still maintaining a healthy, nourishing diet.

Finding Joy in Healthy Eating

The journey towards healthier eating habits should not be one of deprivation and struggle, but rather an opportunity to discover new flavors, textures, and culinary experiences. Finding joy in healthy eating is crucial for long-term success and overall well-being. You probably haven't noticed, but when you genuinely enjoy the food you eat, you're more likely to stick to your healthy eating goals and cultivate a positive relationship with food.

One of the keys to enjoying healthy eating is to focus on abundance rather than restriction. Instead of dwelling on foods you're trying to limit, shift your attention to the wide variety of nutritious foods you can enjoy. Experiment with new fruits, vegetables, whole grains, and lean proteins. Each week, challenge yourself to try a new healthy ingredient or recipe. This approach can turn healthy eating into an exciting culinary adventure rather than a restrictive diet.

Engaging your senses fully while eating is another way to enhance enjoyment. Take time to appreciate the colors, aromas, textures, and flavors of your food. Eat slowly and mindfully, savoring each bite. This not only increases your enjoyment of the meal but also helps you feel more satisfied with smaller portions. Remember, eating is not just about fueling your body; it's also a sensory experience to be savored.

Cooking your own meals is a powerful way to find joy in healthy eating. When you prepare your own food, you have control over the ingredients and cooking methods, allowing you to create meals that are both nutritious and delicious. Cooking can also be a creative outlet and a form of self-care. Experiment with herbs, spices, and healthy cooking techniques to create flavorful dishes that excite your palate.

Don't be afraid to indulge occasionally. A healthy diet can and should include treats in moderation. The key is to savor these indulgences fully and mindfully. When you do enjoy a treat, do so without guilt. Fully immerse yourself in the experience, appreciating every aspect of it. This mindful approach to treats can actually reduce cravings and prevent overindulgence.

Sharing meals with others can greatly enhance the joy of eating. Organize healthy potlucks with friends, cook with family members, or join a cooking club focused on nutritious recipes. The social aspect of eating can make meals more enjoyable and reinforce positive eating habits. Plus, sharing your healthy eating journey with others can provide support and inspiration.

Consider the broader impact of your food choices. Choosing locally sourced, seasonal, or organic ingredients can connect you to your food's origins and the broader food system. This connection can add another layer of enjoyment to your meals, knowing that your choices support local farmers or sustainable practices.

Remember that healthy eating is a journey, not a destination. Be patient with yourself as you develop new habits and preferences. Your tastes will likely change over time, and foods that you once found unappealing might become new favorites. Stay open to trying new things and re-trying foods you previously disliked.

Celebrate your progress and the positive changes you're making. Take note of how eating healthier makes you feel - increased energy, better sleep, improved mood. These positive reinforcements can help you find joy in your healthy eating habits and motivate you to continue.

Lastly, remember that food is just one aspect of a healthy lifestyle. Combine your healthy eating habits with other joyful activities like regular exercise, spending time in nature, or practicing relaxation techniques. This holistic approach to well-being can enhance your overall enjoyment of life, with healthy eating playing a supportive role.

By focusing on the joy and pleasure of healthy eating, you can transform your diet from a series of restrictions into a fulfilling and sustainable lifestyle. Embrace the abundance of nutritious foods available to you, engage all your senses in the eating experience, and celebrate the positive impact of your choices on your health and well-being. With this mindset, healthy eating becomes not just a goal, but a source of daily enjoyment and satisfaction.

Chapter 13: Sustainable Cooking Practices

In the journey towards mastering healthy cooking, it's crucial to consider not only the impact of our food choices on our bodies but also on the environment. Sustainable cooking practices are an integral part of a holistic approach to nutrition and well-being. By adopting eco-friendly methods in the kitchen, you can contribute to a healthier planet while nourishing yourself and your loved ones. This chapter will explore various aspects of sustainable cooking, providing you with practical strategies to reduce your environmental footprint without compromising on the quality or enjoyment of your meals.

Sustainable cooking encompasses a wide range of practices, from minimizing food waste to making conscious decisions about the ingredients you use and the equipment you choose. By implementing these practices, you'll not only reduce your impact on the environment but also often find that you're saving money and creating more flavorful, nutritious meals. As we delve into each aspect of sustainable cooking, you'll discover that many of these practices align perfectly with the principles of healthy eating we've explored throughout this book, "**Viewing Food Through the Lens of Nourishment**"

The concept of sustainability in cooking is not new, but it has gained significant importance in recent years as we've become more aware of the environmental challenges facing our planet. The food system is responsible for about *26%* of global greenhouse gas emissions, with a significant portion coming from agricultural production and food waste[30]. By adopting sustainable cooking practices, you can play a part in reducing these emissions and promoting a more environmentally friendly food system.

Throughout this chapter, we'll explore four key areas of sustainable cooking: reducing food waste, making eco-friendly food choices, embracing seasonal and local eating, and choosing sustainable kitchen equipment. Each of these aspects offers multiple opportunities for you to make a positive impact, and you'll find that many of these practices can be easily integrated into your daily cooking routine. Remember, every small change adds up, and by consistently applying these principles, you'll be contributing to a more sustainable future.

As we explore these sustainable cooking practices, keep in mind that the goal is progress, not perfection. You don't need to implement every suggestion at once. Instead, focus on making gradual changes that you can maintain over time. This approach will help you develop sustainable habits that become second nature, making it easier to stick with these practices in the long run. Let's begin our journey into sustainable cooking by exploring how we can reduce food waste in our kitchens.

Reducing Food Waste in the Kitchen

Food waste is a significant global issue, with approximately one-third of all food produced for human consumption being lost or wasted[31]. This waste not only represents a loss of valuable resources but also contributes to greenhouse gas emissions when it decomposes in landfills. By reducing food waste in your kitchen, you can make a substantial impact on both your environmental footprint and your grocery budget. Let's explore some effective strategies for minimizing food waste in your daily cooking practices.

One of the most impactful ways to reduce food waste is through proper meal planning and shopping. By carefully planning your meals for the week and creating a detailed shopping list, you can avoid overbuying and ensure that you use all the ingredients you purchase. Start by taking inventory of what you already have in your pantry, refrigerator, and freezer. Then, plan your meals around these items, incorporating ingredients that need to be used soon. When shopping, stick to your list and resist the temptation to buy items you don't have a specific plan for. This approach not only reduces waste but also saves you money and time in the long run.

Proper food storage is another crucial aspect of reducing waste. Many foods spoil prematurely due to incorrect storage. Learn the optimal storage conditions for different types of produce, meats, and dairy products. For example, some fruits like apples and bananas release ethylene gas, which can cause nearby produce to ripen and spoil faster. Store these fruits separately from ethylene-sensitive produce like leafy greens. Invest in good quality, airtight containers for storing leftovers and bulk ingredients. Proper storage can significantly extend the life of your food, giving you more time to use it before it spoils.

Understanding expiration dates is also key to reducing food waste. Many people discard food based on the "best by" or "use by" dates without realizing that these are often manufacturer's suggestions for peak quality, not safety. Learn to distinguish between "use by" dates (which are related to safety) and "best before" dates (which are about quality). Use your senses to determine if food is still good to eat – look for signs of spoilage, smell for off odors, and when in doubt, taste a small amount. By being more discerning about expiration dates, you can avoid throwing away perfectly good food.

Another effective strategy is to embrace the concept of "root-to-stem" cooking. This approach involves using as much of each ingredient as possible, including parts that are often discarded. For example, broccoli stems can be peeled and used in stir-fries, carrot tops can be used to make pesto, and citrus peels can be candied or used to infuse water. By finding creative ways to use these often-discarded parts, you not only reduce waste but also add variety and nutrition to your meals. This practice aligns well with traditional cooking methods that emphasized using every part of an ingredient out of necessity and respect for food.

Composting is an excellent way to deal with unavoidable food waste. Even with the best practices, some food waste is inevitable – think vegetable peels, eggshells, and coffee grounds. Instead of sending these to the landfill, start a compost bin. Composting turns food scraps into nutrient-rich soil that can be used in gardens or potted plants. If you don't have space for a compost bin, look for community composting programs in your area. Many cities now offer food waste collection services or have community gardens that accept compost donations.

Preserving excess produce is another effective way to reduce waste while extending your enjoyment of seasonal foods. When you have more fruits or vegetables than you can use before they spoil, consider freezing, canning, or fermenting them. Freezing is particularly easy and works well for many fruits and vegetables. Blanch vegetables briefly before freezing to preserve their color and texture. Canning requires more equipment and knowledge but allows you to preserve a wide variety of foods for long-term storage. Fermentation not only preserves food but also enhances its nutritional value and flavor.

Lastly, get creative with leftovers. Instead of letting leftover ingredients or meals languish in the refrigerator, plan to use them in new dishes. Leftover roasted vegetables can be blended into soups or added to frittatas. Cooked grains can be transformed into salads or stir-fries. By viewing leftovers as ingredients for new meals rather than as less desirable repeats, you can reduce waste and add variety to your diet. Keep a "use first" bin in your refrigerator for ingredients that need to be used soon and challenge yourself to create meals using these items.

Implementing these strategies for reducing food waste in your kitchen can have a significant impact on your environmental footprint and your budget. Start by focusing on one or two areas where you feel you can make the most immediate impact and gradually incorporate more practices over time. Remember, every bit of food saved from the landfill is a step towards a more sustainable future.

Making Eco-Friendly Food Choices

The food choices we make have a profound impact on the environment. From the way food is produced to how it's packaged and transported, every step in the food system can contribute to or mitigate environmental issues. By making eco-friendly food choices, you can significantly reduce your carbon footprint and support more sustainable food production practices. Let's explore some key strategies for making environmentally conscious decisions in your food purchases and consumption.

One of the most impactful changes you can make is to reduce your consumption of animal products, particularly red meat. Livestock, especially cattle, are major contributors to greenhouse gas emissions due to their methane production and the large amounts of land and water required for their feed[32]. Consider adopting a more plant-based diet, even if only for a few meals a week. This doesn't mean you have to become fully vegetarian or vegan – even small reductions in meat consumption can make a significant difference. When you do choose to eat meat, opt for poultry or fish, which generally have a lower environmental impact than beef or lamb.

Choosing sustainably sourced seafood is another important aspect of eco-friendly eating. Overfishing and destructive fishing practices have led to the depletion of many fish populations and damage to marine ecosystems. When buying seafood, look for certifications from organizations like the Marine Stewardship Council (MSC) or the Aquaculture Stewardship Council (ASC), which indicate that the fish has been sourced using sustainable practices. You can also use seafood guides provided by organizations like the Monterey Bay Aquarium's Seafood Watch program to make informed choices about which species to buy and which to avoid.

Opting for organic produce when possible is another way to support more environmentally friendly farming practices. Organic farming methods typically use fewer synthetic pesticides and fertilizers, which can have harmful effects on soil health, water quality, and biodiversity. While organic produce can be more expensive, you can prioritize organic for the "Dirty Dozen" – a list of fruits and vegetables that tend to have the highest pesticide residues when grown conventionally. These include strawberries, spinach, kale, nectarines, and apples, among others. For produce that's less likely to retain pesticide residues, such as avocados, sweet corn, and pineapples, conventional options may be a more budget-friendly choice.

Reducing your reliance on processed and packaged foods is another effective way to make more eco-friendly food choices. Highly processed foods often come with excessive packaging, which contributes to plastic waste. They also typically require more energy to produce and transport than whole foods. By focusing your diet on whole, minimally processed ingredients, you not only reduce packaging waste but also tend to eat a more nutritious diet. When you do buy packaged foods, look for options with minimal or recyclable packaging.

Choosing foods with minimal packaging or bringing your own containers for bulk purchases can significantly reduce your plastic waste. Many grocery stores now offer bulk bins for items like grains, nuts, and dried fruits. By bringing your own reusable containers or bags to fill from these bins, you can avoid single-use plastic packaging altogether. For produce, skip the plastic bags and either carry items loose or use reusable produce bags. When shopping for staples like olive oil or vinegar, look for brands that use glass bottles rather than plastic, as glass is more easily recycled and doesn't leach chemicals into the food.

Supporting local food systems is another important aspect of eco-friendly eating. Locally produced food often has a lower carbon footprint due to reduced transportation distances. Additionally, supporting local farmers and producers helps maintain agricultural diversity and can contribute to the economic resilience of your community. Look for farmers' markets in your area, join a Community Supported Agriculture (CSA) program, or seek out locally produced items at your grocery store. Many regions also have food co-ops that prioritize local and sustainable products.

Consider growing some of your own food, even if you only have a small space. Herbs, lettuce, and cherry tomatoes can be grown in pots on a balcony or windowsill. If you have a yard, you might be able to grow a wider variety of vegetables. Growing your own food not only reduces the environmental impact of transportation and packaging but also gives you a deeper appreciation for the food production process. It can also be a rewarding and educational experience, especially if you have children.

When it comes to beverages, tap water is generally the most environmentally friendly choice. If you're concerned about water quality, invest in a good water filter rather than relying on bottled water. For other beverages, choose those in recyclable containers and avoid single-use plastic bottles whenever possible. If you enjoy coffee or tea, consider using a reusable filter or loose-leaf tea instead of single-use pods or tea bags, many of which contain plastic.

Lastly, be mindful of food trends and their environmental impact. For example, while foods like quinoa and avocados are nutritious, their increased global popularity has led to environmental and social issues in some producing regions. This doesn't mean you need to avoid these foods entirely, but being aware of these impacts can help you make more informed decisions about how often to include them in your diet.

By implementing these eco-friendly food choices, you can significantly reduce the environmental impact of your diet. Remember, every choice matters, and even small changes can add up to make a big difference over time. As you become more aware of the environmental implications of your food choices, you'll likely find that making eco-friendly decisions becomes second nature, contributing to both your health and the health of the planet.

Embracing Seasonal and Local Eating

Embracing seasonal and local eating is a powerful way to enhance the sustainability of your diet while also enjoying fresher, more flavorful food. This approach to eating aligns closely with natural growing cycles and supports local food systems, reducing the environmental impact of long-distance transportation and storage. Let's explore the benefits of seasonal and local eating and how you can incorporate these practices into your cooking routine.

Eating seasonally means consuming fruits and vegetables at the time of year when they naturally ripen in your local area. This practice has several environmental benefits. Seasonal produce typically requires less artificial input to grow, such as heated greenhouses or extensive pesticide use, as it's being cultivated in its natural growing season. Additionally, seasonal eating often correlates with local eating, which means food travels shorter distances from farm to table, reducing transportation-related emissions. A study by the University of Michigan found that the average American meal travels about 1,500 miles from farm to plate, contributing significantly to greenhouse gas emissions[33].

Beyond the environmental benefits, seasonal eating offers nutritional advantages. Fruits and vegetables picked at peak ripeness tend to have higher nutrient content compared to those harvested early for long-distance shipping. For example, a study published in the Journal of Agricultural and Food Chemistry found that broccoli grown in season had higher levels of vitamin *C* and flavonoids compared to broccoli grown out of season[34]. Additionally, seasonal produce is often fresher and more flavorful, which can make your meals more enjoyable and may encourage you to eat more fruits and vegetables overall.

To embrace seasonal eating, start by familiarizing yourself with your local growing seasons. This can vary depending on your geographic location. Many local agriculture departments or extension offices provide guides to seasonal produce in your area. You can also observe what's abundant and inexpensive at your local farmers' market or grocery store, as this often reflects what's in season. Create a seasonal eating calendar for your region and use it to plan your meals and shopping.

Local eating goes hand in hand with seasonal eating and offers additional benefits. By purchasing food grown or produced locally, you're supporting your local economy and helping to maintain agricultural diversity in your region. Local food systems also tend to be more transparent, allowing you to learn more about how your food is produced and potentially even visit the farms where your food is grown. This connection to your food source can lead to a greater appreciation for the food you eat and the work that goes into producing it.

To incorporate more local foods into your diet, seek out farmers' markets, farm stands, and Community Supported Agriculture (CSA) programs in your area. Many grocery stores also highlight locally sourced products. When shopping, look for labels indicating local origin, or ask store staff about local options. Remember that "local" can mean different things depending on where you live – in some areas, it might mean within *100* miles, while in others, it could encompass a wider region.

Adapting your cooking to seasonal and local eating can require some creativity and flexibility. Instead of starting with a recipe and then shopping for ingredients, try reversing the process: see what's available seasonally and locally, then plan your meals around these ingredients. This approach can lead to more varied and interesting meals as you experiment with new ingredients and combinations. It can also help you develop a deeper understanding of the natural rhythms of food production in your area.

Preserving seasonal abundance is another important aspect of embracing seasonal eating. When local produce is at its peak and plentiful, consider preserving some for use later in the year. This could involve freezing, canning, pickling, or fermenting. For example, you might freeze berries at the height of summer for use in smoothies during winter, or make tomato sauce to can when tomatoes are abundant in late summer. These preservation techniques allow you to enjoy local, seasonal flavors year-round while reducing your reliance on out-of-season produce.

It's important to note that strict adherence to local and seasonal eating may not be practical or desirable for everyone. In some climates, a purely local diet could be very limited during certain times of the year. Additionally, some non-local foods may have important nutritional or cultural significance in your diet. The goal is to increase your consumption of seasonal and local foods where possible, rather than to eliminate all non-local foods. Even small shifts towards more seasonal and local eating can have positive impacts.

Embracing seasonal and local eating is a journey that can deepen your connection to your food and your local environment. It encourages a more diverse diet, supports local food systems, and often results in fresher, more flavorful meals. As you become more attuned to the rhythms of local food production, you may find that your cooking becomes more creative and satisfying. Remember, every meal is an opportunity to make choices that support both your health and the health of your local food system.

Choosing Sustainable Kitchen Equipment

The equipment we use in our kitchens plays a significant role in the overall sustainability of our cooking practices. From the energy efficiency of our appliances to the materials used in our cookware and utensils, every item in our kitchen has an environmental footprint. By making informed choices about our kitchen equipment, we can reduce energy consumption, minimize waste, and support more sustainable manufacturing practices. Let's explore some key considerations for choosing sustainable kitchen equipment and how to make the most eco-friendly decisions for your cooking needs.

When it comes to major appliances like refrigerators, ovens, and dishwashers, energy efficiency should be a top priority. Look for appliances with high energy efficiency ratings, such as those certified by ENERGY STAR in the United States. These appliances use less energy to operate, which not only reduces your environmental impact but also saves you money on utility bills over time. For example, ENERGY STAR certified refrigerators use about *15%* less energy than non-certified models, while ENERGY STAR dishwashers are *12%* more energy efficient and *30%* more water efficient than standard models[35].

When choosing cookware, consider both the materials used and their durability. Cast iron and stainless steel are excellent choices for sustainable cookware. These materials are long-lasting, can withstand high temperatures, and are recyclable at the end of their life. Cast iron, in particular, can last for generations if properly cared for. While non-stick cookware can be convenient, many traditional non-stick coatings contain chemicals that can be harmful to the environment and potentially to human health. If you do opt for non-stick cookware, look for options with ceramic coatings, which are generally considered more environmentally friendly.

For smaller appliances and kitchen tools, prioritize multi-functional items to reduce the overall number of gadgets in your kitchen. For example, a high-quality blender can serve as a food processor, smoothie maker, and even a grain mill. This approach not only saves space but also reduces the resources required to manufacture and eventually dispose of multiple single-use appliances. When purchasing small appliances, look for those with durable construction and replaceable parts, which can extend their lifespan and reduce waste.

Consider the environmental impact of disposable kitchen items and look for reusable alternatives. Replace paper towels with cloth napkins or reusable kitchen towels. Swap plastic wrap and aluminum foil for reusable silicone food covers or beeswax wraps. Use glass or stainless steel food storage containers instead of disposable plastic bags. While these reusable options may have a higher upfront cost, they save money in the long run and significantly reduce waste.

When it comes to utensils and cutting boards, opt for materials like bamboo or sustainably harvested wood. These materials are renewable and biodegradable. Avoid plastic utensils, which can leach chemicals into food and are difficult to recycle. For cutting boards, end-grain wood boards are particularly durable and can last for many years with proper care. If you do need to use plastic for certain tasks, choose high-quality, durable plastic that won't need frequent replacement.

Consider the packaging and manufacturing practices of the companies you buy from. Look for brands that use minimal, recyclable packaging and those that have transparent sustainability practices. Some companies now use recycled materials in their products or have take-back programs for recycling old equipment. Supporting these companies encourages more sustainable practices across the industry.

Proper maintenance of your kitchen equipment is crucial for sustainability. Regular cleaning and care can significantly extend the life of your appliances and cookware, reducing the need for replacements. Learn the correct care techniques for different materials – for example, seasoning cast iron pans or sharpening knives regularly. When appliances do break, consider repair before replacement. Many appliances can be fixed, often for less than the cost of a new item, and this approach keeps functional components out of landfills.

For items that you only use occasionally, consider borrowing or renting rather than buying. Many communities have kitchen equipment libraries or tool-sharing programs. This approach not only reduces the resources needed to manufacture new items but also saves you money and storage space. It's particularly useful for specialized equipment like canning supplies or large roasting pans that you might only use a few times a year.

When you do need to dispose of kitchen equipment, do so responsibly. Many materials, including metals and some plastics, can be recycled. For electronic appliances, look for e-waste recycling programs in your area. Some retailers and manufacturers also offer take-back programs for old appliances. Donating usable items to charity shops or community organizations is another way to extend the life of kitchen equipment you no longer need.

Lastly, remember that the most sustainable kitchen equipment is often that which you already own. Before purchasing new items, assess what you have and whether it meets your needs. Sometimes, creative use of existing tools can eliminate the need for new purchases. When you do buy new equipment, choose high-quality items that will last for many years, reducing the overall environmental impact of your kitchen setup.

By making thoughtful choices about your kitchen equipment, you can significantly reduce the environmental impact of your cooking practices. From energy-efficient appliances to durable, sustainable materials, every choice contributes to a more eco-friendly kitchen. Remember, sustainability in the kitchen is not just about what you cook, but also about how you cook and the tools you use to do it.

Conclusion

As we reach the culmination of this culinary journey through "*Viewing Food Through the Lens of Nourishment:* A Comprehensive Guide to Mastering Healthy Cooking," it's time to reflect on the transformative power of healthy cooking and the profound impact it can have on your overall well-being. Throughout this book, you've explored a wealth of knowledge, techniques, and recipes that have equipped you with the tools to revolutionize your approach to food and nutrition. The journey to mastering healthy cooking is ongoing, and the skills you've acquired are just the beginning of a lifelong adventure in nourishing your body and delighting your taste buds.

The path to a healthier lifestyle through cooking is not always straightforward, but it is undoubtedly rewarding. By embracing the principles and practices outlined in this guide, you've taken significant steps towards improving your health, enhancing your culinary skills, and developing a more mindful relationship with food. Remember that every meal you prepare is an opportunity to nourish your body, express your creativity, and share love with those around you. As you continue to apply the knowledge gained from this book, you'll find that healthy cooking becomes not just a habit, but a joyful and integral part of your daily life.

The journey of healthy cooking is one of continuous discovery and growth. As you experiment with new ingredients, perfect your techniques, and create your own signature dishes, you'll find that your confidence in the kitchen grows alongside your health and vitality. The recipes and methods you've learned are not rigid rules, but flexible guidelines that you can adapt to suit your tastes, dietary needs, and lifestyle. The true essence of mastering healthy cooking lies not just in following recipes, but in understanding the principles behind them and having the confidence to innovate and make them your own.

As you move forward, remember that small, consistent changes can lead to significant improvements in your health and well-being. Every time you choose whole foods over processed alternatives, experiment with a new vegetable, or try a healthier cooking method, you're taking a step towards a more vibrant and energetic life. The journey of healthy cooking is not about perfection, but about progress and the joy of learning and growing. Embrace the process, celebrate your successes, and learn from your culinary experiments – both the triumphs and the occasional mishaps.

In this conclusion, we'll reflect on the key aspects of embracing a healthy cooking lifestyle and explore ways to continue your culinary education. These final thoughts will help solidify your commitment to healthy cooking and provide inspiration for your ongoing journey in the kitchen and beyond.

As we conclude this comprehensive guide to mastering healthy cooking, it's important to recognize the significant journey you've undertaken. You've not only acquired a wealth of knowledge about nutrition, ingredients, and cooking techniques, but you've also embarked on a transformative path towards better health and well-being. The skills and insights you've gained are powerful tools that will serve you well in your ongoing pursuit of a healthier lifestyle.

Remember that the essence of healthy cooking lies not in perfection, but in the joy of creating nourishing meals that support your health goals and delight your senses. As you continue to apply the principles and techniques learned in this book, you'll find that healthy cooking becomes an integral and enjoyable part of your daily life. The journey doesn't end here – it's a continuous process of learning, experimenting, and growing.

Embrace the challenges and celebrate the successes as you continue to explore the world of healthy cooking. Let your curiosity guide you to new ingredients, flavors, and techniques. Share your passion with others, and draw inspiration from the vast community of health-conscious cooks around the world. With each meal you prepare, you're not just feeding your body; you're nurturing your overall well-being and contributing to a healthier, more sustainable world.

As you close this book and step into your kitchen, do so with confidence, creativity, and enthusiasm. The journey of healthy cooking is one of endless possibilities and discoveries. May your culinary adventures be filled with delicious, nutritious meals that nourish your body, mind, and spirit. Here's to your health, your happiness, and the wonderful meals that lie ahead. Happy cooking!

Embracing a Healthy Cooking Lifestyle

Adopting a healthy cooking lifestyle is about more than just preparing nutritious meals; it's a holistic approach that encompasses mindful eating, sustainable practices, and a positive relationship with food. As you've learned throughout this book, healthy cooking is a powerful tool for transforming your overall well-being. It's about nourishing your body with wholesome ingredients, experimenting with flavors and textures, and finding joy in the process of creating meals that are both delicious and nutritious. By embracing this lifestyle, you're not just changing what's on your plate – you're changing your entire approach to food and health.

One of the most significant aspects of a healthy cooking lifestyle is the shift in mindset it brings. Instead of viewing food merely as fuel or falling into the trap of restrictive dieting, you've learned to see food as a source of nourishment, pleasure, and connection. This perspective allows you to make choices that are both satisfying and beneficial for your health. You've discovered that healthy eating doesn't mean sacrificing flavor or enjoyment; rather, it's about enhancing your culinary experiences with nutrient-dense ingredients and creative cooking techniques. This positive approach to food can have far-reaching effects on your physical health, mental well-being, and overall quality of life.

Incorporating the principles of nutrition you've learned into your daily cooking routine is a cornerstone of the healthy cooking lifestyle. You now understand the importance of balancing macronutrients, incorporating a variety of colorful fruits and vegetables, and choosing whole grains and lean proteins. This knowledge empowers you to make informed decisions about your meals, ensuring that each dish you create contributes to your overall health goals. Remember that nutrition is not about perfection, but about making consistent, informed choices that nourish your body and support your well-being.

The skills and techniques you've acquired throughout this journey are invaluable tools in your healthy cooking arsenal. From mastering various cooking methods that preserve nutrients to learning how to enhance flavors naturally, you've expanded your culinary repertoire in ways that support your health goals. These skills allow you to transform simple, whole ingredients into delicious meals that rival any restaurant dish. As you continue to practice and refine these techniques, you'll find that healthy cooking becomes second nature, making it easier to maintain your commitment to a nutritious diet.

Meal planning and preparation have become essential components of your healthy cooking lifestyle. By taking the time to plan your meals, shop for ingredients, and prepare food in advance, you've set yourself up for success in maintaining a healthy diet even during busy times. This proactive approach not only ensures that you have nutritious meals readily available but also reduces stress and saves time during the week. As you continue to refine your meal planning strategies, you'll find that it becomes an enjoyable and rewarding part of your routine, rather than a chore.

The concept of mindful eating is another crucial aspect of the healthy cooking lifestyle you've embraced. By paying attention to your food choices, savoring each bite, and listening to your body's hunger and fullness cues, you've developed a more conscious and enjoyable relationship with food. This mindful approach extends beyond the act of eating to encompass the entire process of meal preparation. As you chop vegetables, mix ingredients, and cook your meals, you're fully present in the moment, appreciating the colors, textures, and aromas of your food. This mindfulness not only enhances your enjoyment of cooking and eating but also helps you make more intentional and health-conscious choices.

Sustainability has become an integral part of your healthy cooking lifestyle. You've learned the importance of reducing food waste, choosing seasonal and local ingredients, and making eco-friendly decisions in the kitchen. These practices not only benefit the environment but also often result in fresher, more flavorful meals. By aligning your cooking habits with sustainable principles, you're contributing to a healthier planet while nourishing your body – a truly holistic approach to well-being.

As you continue to embrace this healthy cooking lifestyle, remember that it's a journey of continuous learning and adaptation. Your tastes, nutritional needs, and life circumstances may change over time, and your approach to healthy cooking can evolve accordingly. Stay curious, be open to trying new ingredients and techniques, and don't be afraid to experiment in the kitchen. The flexibility and creativity you've developed will serve you well as you navigate these changes and continue to grow as a healthy cook.

Finally, sharing your passion for healthy cooking with others can be an incredibly rewarding aspect of this lifestyle. Whether you're cooking for family and friends, exchanging recipes with colleagues, or inspiring others through social media, your enthusiasm for nutritious and delicious food can have a positive ripple effect. By sharing your knowledge and creations, you're not only reinforcing your own commitment to healthy cooking but also potentially inspiring others to embark on their own culinary health journeys.

Embracing a healthy cooking lifestyle is a powerful commitment to your well-being that extends far beyond the kitchen. It's a choice to nourish your body, mind, and spirit through the food you prepare and consume. As you continue on this path, take pride in the positive changes you've made and the skills you've developed. Your journey in healthy cooking is an ongoing adventure – one that promises continued growth, discovery, and a lifetime of delicious, nutritious meals.

Continuing Your Culinary Education

The journey of mastering healthy cooking is a lifelong adventure, filled with opportunities for growth, discovery, and refinement of your skills. As you've progressed through this book, you've built a solid foundation of knowledge and techniques. However, the world of culinary arts and nutrition is vast and ever-evolving, offering endless possibilities for expanding your expertise. Continuing your culinary education is not just about learning new recipes or techniques; it's about deepening your understanding of food, nutrition, and the art of cooking. This ongoing learning process will keep your healthy cooking journey exciting, inspiring, and rewarding for years to come.

One of the most effective ways to continue your culinary education is to stay curious and open to new experiences. Challenge yourself to try a new ingredient or cooking method each week or month. This could mean experimenting with an unfamiliar grain, learning to prepare a vegetable you've never cooked before, or mastering a new healthy cooking technique. By regularly stepping out of your comfort zone, you'll expand your culinary repertoire and discover new flavors and textures to incorporate into your meals. This approach not only enhances your cooking skills but also ensures that your diet remains varied and nutritionally diverse.

Keeping up with the latest nutritional research and dietary guidelines is another crucial aspect of continuing your culinary education. The field of nutrition is dynamic, with new studies and recommendations emerging regularly. Stay informed by following reputable nutrition websites, subscribing to health and cooking magazines, or attending workshops and seminars on nutrition and healthy cooking. This ongoing education will help you make informed decisions about your food choices and cooking methods, ensuring that your approach to healthy cooking remains grounded in current scientific understanding.

Exploring cuisines from different cultures can be an incredibly enriching way to expand your culinary horizons. Each culture has its own unique ingredients, flavor combinations, and cooking techniques, many of which align beautifully with the principles of healthy cooking. By delving into various world cuisines, you'll discover new ways to prepare familiar ingredients and encounter entirely new foods to incorporate into your diet. This cultural exploration not only broadens your culinary skills but also adds excitement and variety to your meals, making healthy eating a continually engaging experience.

Investing in your culinary education through cooking classes or workshops can provide structured learning experiences and hands-on practice. Look for classes that focus on healthy cooking techniques, specific cuisines, or specialized dietary approaches. Many cooking schools and community centers offer courses on topics like plant-based cooking, gluten-free baking, or cooking for specific health conditions. These classes not only teach you new skills but also provide opportunities to connect with other health-conscious cooks and share ideas and experiences.

In today's digital age, online resources offer a wealth of opportunities for continuing your culinary education. Explore cooking blogs, social channels, and social media accounts dedicated to healthy cooking for inspiration, recipes, and tips. Many professional chefs and nutritionists share their knowledge through online platforms, offering everything from quick cooking hacks to in-depth tutorials on advanced techniques. Engaging with these online communities can also provide support and motivation as you continue your healthy cooking journey.

Cookbooks remain an invaluable resource for expanding your culinary knowledge. While this book has provided a comprehensive foundation, exploring other cookbooks focused on healthy cooking, specific cuisines, or particular dietary approaches can offer new perspectives and ideas. Look for cookbooks that not only provide recipes but also explain the principles behind healthy cooking and offer insights into ingredient selection and nutritional benefits. Reading cookbooks can be an enjoyable way to discover new flavor combinations, learn about ingredient substitutions, and gain inspiration for your own culinary creations.

Participating in cooking challenges or joining a cooking club can add an element of fun and community to your ongoing culinary education. These activities encourage you to try new recipes, work with unfamiliar ingredients, and push your culinary boundaries. They also provide opportunities to share your creations, get feedback, and learn from others. Whether it's a virtual cooking challenge or a local healthy cooking club, these experiences can keep you motivated and engaged in your healthy cooking journey.

As you continue to develop your skills, consider keeping a cooking journal or blog to document your experiences, recipes, and learnings. This practice not only helps you track your progress and remember successful recipes but also encourages reflection on your cooking process. Writing about your culinary adventures can deepen your understanding of ingredients, techniques, and flavor combinations. It's also a great way to share your knowledge and inspire others who are interested in healthy cooking.

Remember that continuing your culinary education isn't just about accumulating knowledge – it's about applying what you learn to create healthier, more delicious meals. As you discover new information or techniques, challenge yourself to incorporate them into your cooking routine. Experiment with adapting your favorite recipes to make them healthier or create entirely new dishes based on the principles you've learned. This practical application of knowledge is where true learning and growth occur.

Finally, don't underestimate the value of teaching others as a way of deepening your own understanding. As you become more confident in your healthy cooking skills, share your knowledge with friends, family, or even in community settings. Teaching others not only reinforces your own learning but also often leads to new insights and perspectives. It's a rewarding way to contribute to your community while continuing to grow in your own culinary journey.

Continuing your culinary education is a lifelong commitment that will enrich your healthy cooking journey in countless ways. By staying curious, exploring new cuisines and techniques, engaging with culinary communities, and applying your knowledge creatively, you'll ensure that your approach to healthy cooking remains fresh, exciting, and aligned with your evolving tastes and nutritional needs. Remember, every meal is an opportunity to learn and grow. Embrace the journey with enthusiasm, and let your passion for healthy cooking continue to flourish and inspire both you and all of those who are around you.

Appendix

Welcome to the Appendix of "*Viewing Food Through the Lens of Nourishment*: A Comprehensive Guide to Mastering Healthy Cooking." This section serves as a valuable reference tool to support your culinary journey. Here, you'll find essential information that will help you navigate the world of healthy cooking with greater ease and precision. The Appendix is designed to complement the main chapters of the book, providing quick access to practical information that you'll likely refer to time and again as you experiment with new recipes and techniques.

The Appendix is divided into two main sections: Measurement Conversions and Cooking Times for Common Ingredients. These resources are crucial for ensuring accuracy in your cooking, which is particularly important when you're focusing on creating nutritionally balanced meals. Whether you're adapting a recipe from a different measurement system or trying to perfect the cooking time for a new ingredient, these sections will serve as your go-to guide.

As you progress through your healthy cooking journey, you'll find that having this information readily available will boost your confidence in the kitchen. It will allow you to focus more on the creative aspects of cooking, knowing that you have reliable reference points for the technical details. Remember, cooking is both an art and a science, and this Appendix aims to support you in mastering both aspects.

Let's dive into each section of the Appendix, exploring how these tools can enhance your cooking experience and help you achieve consistent, delicious results in your healthy meal preparations.

Measurement Conversions

Accurate measurements are the foundation of successful cooking, especially when it comes to healthy recipes where nutritional balance is key. This section provides comprehensive conversion tables for various units of measurement commonly used in cooking. Whether you're working with a recipe that uses metric or imperial measurements, or you need to adjust serving sizes, these conversions will ensure your ingredients are properly proportioned.

Let's start with volume conversions, which are essential for liquid ingredients and many dry goods. Here's a basic conversion table for common volume measurements:

- *1* cup = *8* fluid ounces = *237* milliliters
- *1* tablespoon = *3* teaspoons = *15* milliliters
- *1* fluid ounce = *2* tablespoons = *30* milliliters
- *1* pint = *2* cups = *473* milliliters
- *1* quart = *4* cups = *946* milliliters
- *1* gallon = *16* cups = *3.78* liters

For dry ingredients, weight measurements often provide more accuracy than volume. Here's a conversion table for common weight measurements:

- *1* ounce = *28.35* grams
- *1* pound = *16* ounces = *453.6* grams
- *1* kilogram = *2.2* pounds = *1,000* grams

When it comes to temperature conversions, which are crucial for baking and ensuring food safety, use these formulas:

- Fahrenheit to Celsius: $(°F - 32) \times 5/9 = °C$
- Celsius to Fahrenheit: $(°C \times 9/5) + 32 = °F$

Common temperature conversions include:

- *32°F = 0°C* (freezing point of water)
- *212°F = 100°C* (boiling point of water at sea level)
- *350°F = 175°C* (common baking temperature)
- *375°F = 190°C* (medium-high oven temperature)
- *400°F = 200°C* (high oven temperature)

Understanding these conversions will allow you to adapt recipes from various sources and cuisines, expanding your repertoire of healthy dishes. It's particularly useful when working with international recipes or when scaling recipes up or down to accommodate different serving sizes.

For ingredients that are commonly used in small quantities, such as spices or leavening agents, it's helpful to know these conversions:

- *1/4* teaspoon = *1.25* milliliters
- *1/2* teaspoon = *2.5* milliliters
- *1* teaspoon = *5* milliliters
- *1* tablespoon = *15* milliliters = *3* teaspoons

When working with fresh produce, conversions can be less precise due to variations in size and density. However, these general guidelines can be helpful:

- *1* medium onion = about *1* cup chopped
- *1* medium bell pepper = about *1* cup chopped
- *1* medium apple = about *1* cup sliced
- *1* cup of leafy greens = about *2* ounces by weight

Remember that while these conversions are generally accurate, slight variations can occur due to factors such as ingredient density, humidity, and even altitude. When precision is crucial, especially in baking or when calculating nutritional information, it's best to use a kitchen scale for the most accurate measurements.

As you become more comfortable with these conversions, you'll find it easier to experiment with recipes, substitute ingredients, and create your own healthy dishes. This flexibility is key to maintaining a varied and enjoyable healthy diet, allowing you to adapt to seasonal ingredients and personal preferences while still maintaining the nutritional balance that is central to healthy cooking.

Cooking Times for Common Ingredients

Understanding the appropriate cooking times for various ingredients is crucial in healthy cooking. Proper cooking ensures that foods retain their nutritional value, achieve the right texture, and develop optimal flavor. Overcooking can lead to loss of nutrients and poor texture, while undercooking may result in food safety issues and unpalatable dishes. This section provides a comprehensive guide to cooking times for common ingredients, helping you achieve perfect results every time.

Let's start with vegetables, which form the cornerstone of many healthy meals. Cooking times can vary based on the method used (steaming, roasting, sautéing, etc.) and the size of the cut. Here's a general guide for steaming vegetables, which is one of the healthiest cooking methods as it preserves nutrients:

- Asparagus: *5-7* minutes
- Broccoli florets: *5-7* minutes
- Carrots (sliced): *7-10* minutes
- Cauliflower florets: *5-7* minutes
- Green beans: *5-7* minutes
- Leafy greens (kale, spinach): *3-5* minutes
- Peas: *3-5* minutes
- Potatoes (cubed): *12-15* minutes
- Sweet potatoes (cubed): *10-12* minutes
- Zucchini (sliced): *5-7* minutes

For roasting vegetables, which can enhance flavor through caramelization, typical oven temperatures range from *375°F* to *425°F* (*190°C* to *220°C*). Here are some general roasting times:

- Asparagus: *10-15* minutes
- Brussels sprouts (halved): *20-25* minutes
- Carrots (chopped): *25-30* minutes

- Cauliflower florets: *20-25* minutes
- Eggplant (cubed): *20-25* minutes
- Potatoes (cubed): *25-30* minutes
- Sweet potatoes (cubed): *20-25* minutes
- Winter squash (cubed): *25-30* minutes

When it comes to grains and legumes, cooking times can vary significantly. Here's a guide for cooking times, assuming the grains or legumes have been soaked overnight where appropriate:

- Brown rice: *40-45* minutes
- Quinoa: *15-20* minutes
- Barley: *40-50* minutes
- Lentils (green or brown): *20-30* minutes
- Chickpeas: *1-2* hours
- Black beans: *1-1.5* hours
- Millet: *20-25* minutes
- Steel-cut oats: *20-30* minutes

For proteins, cooking times can vary based on the cut, thickness, and desired doneness. Here are some guidelines for common proteins, assuming medium heat for stovetop cooking and *350°F* (*175°C*) for oven cooking:

- Chicken breast (boneless, skinless): *6-8* minutes per side on stovetop, *25-30* minutes in oven
- Fish fillet (*1*-inch thick): *4-5* minutes per side on stovetop, *15-20* minutes in oven
- Tofu (*1*-inch cubes): *5-7* minutes per side when pan-frying
- Tempeh (sliced): *3-4* minutes per side when pan-frying
- Eggs (boiled): *6* minutes for soft-boiled, *10* minutes for hard-boiled

It's important to note that these times are general guidelines and may need to be adjusted based on factors such as the specific recipe, the size and thickness of the ingredients, and your particular cooking equipment. Always use visual cues and, where appropriate, a food thermometer to ensure that foods are cooked to safe temperatures.

For baking, which often involves combining multiple ingredients, cooking times can be more complex. Here are some general guidelines for common baked goods:

- Muffins: *18-20* minutes at *375°F (190°C)*
- Cookies: *8-12* minutes at *350°F (175°C)*
- Bread loaf: *30-40* minutes at *350°F (175°C)*
- Whole grain pizza crust: *12-15* minutes at *450°F (230°C)*

Remember that altitude, humidity, and variations in oven performance can all affect cooking times. It's always a good idea to check your food a few minutes before the suggested cooking time is up, and to use visual cues (like golden-brown color for baked goods) or internal temperature checks for meats to determine doneness.

As you gain experience with healthy cooking, you'll develop an intuitive sense of cooking times for your favorite ingredients. This will allow you to multitask more efficiently in the kitchen, timing different components of your meal to finish cooking simultaneously. The ability to cook ingredients properly is a fundamental skill in healthy cooking, ensuring that you get the most nutritional benefit and best flavor from your ingredients.

Glossary

Welcome to the glossary section of "*Viewing Food Through the Lens of Nourishment:* A Comprehensive Guide to Mastering Healthy Cooking." This comprehensive glossary is designed to be your go-to reference for understanding the terminology, techniques, and concepts discussed throughout the book. Whether you're a novice cook or an experienced culinary enthusiast, this glossary will help clarify any unfamiliar terms and reinforce your understanding of key concepts in healthy cooking and nutrition.

The terms in this glossary are arranged alphabetically for easy navigation. Each entry provides a clear and concise definition, often accompanied by additional context or examples to enhance your understanding. As you progress through your healthy cooking journey, you may find yourself referring back to this glossary frequently to refresh your knowledge or gain deeper insights into specific topics.

Remember, cooking is both an art and a science, and the language used in culinary circles can sometimes be complex or technical. This glossary aims to demystify that language, making it accessible and understandable for everyone. By familiarizing yourself with these terms, you'll be better equipped to follow recipes, understand nutritional information, and communicate effectively about food and cooking.

Let's dive into the world of culinary terminology and nutritional concepts that will empower you to become a more knowledgeable and confident healthy cook.

A

Al dente: An Italian term meaning "to the tooth," used to describe pasta or vegetables that are cooked until they are firm to the bite but not soft or mushy. This cooking technique helps retain nutrients and texture in foods.

Antioxidants: Compounds found in foods that help protect your body's cells from damage caused by free radicals. Antioxidants are abundant in many fruits, vegetables, and other plant-based foods, and are associated with numerous health benefits, including reduced risk of chronic diseases.

Aromatics: Vegetables, herbs, and spices that are cooked to release their flavors and aromas, forming the base of many dishes. Common aromatics include onions, garlic, ginger, and celery. Using aromatics is a great way to add depth and complexity to dishes without relying on excessive salt or fat.

B

Blanching: A cooking technique where food, typically vegetables or fruits, is briefly immersed in boiling water and then quickly cooled in ice water. This process helps preserve color, texture, and nutritional value, making it an excellent method for preparing vegetables for freezing or further cooking.

Braising: A cooking method that involves first searing food at a high temperature, then cooking it slowly in a small amount of liquid in a covered pot. This technique is particularly useful for tougher cuts of meat, as it helps break down connective tissues, resulting in tender, flavorful dishes.

Broiling: A cooking method that uses direct heat from above to cook food quickly at high temperatures. Broiling can be an excellent way to cook lean proteins and vegetables, as it requires little to no added fat and helps retain moisture in foods.

C

Caramelization: The process of heating sugars until they break down and turn brown, producing complex flavors and aromas. This technique is often used to enhance the natural sweetness and depth of flavor in vegetables and fruits without adding extra sugar.

Chia seeds: Small, nutrient-dense seeds that are high in fiber, protein, and omega-*3* fatty acids. Chia seeds can absorb liquid and form a gel-like consistency, making them useful in recipes as a thickening agent or egg substitute in vegan baking.

Cruciferous vegetables: A family of vegetables that includes broccoli, cauliflower, Brussels sprouts, and kale. These vegetables are known for their high nutrient content, including vitamins, minerals, and beneficial plant compounds that may help reduce the risk of certain cancers and other chronic diseases.

D

Deglaze: The process of adding liquid (such as broth, wine, or water) to a pan after sautéing or roasting to loosen and dissolve the flavorful browned bits stuck to the bottom. This technique is used to create flavorful sauces and gravies without relying on heavy cream or excessive fat.

Dietary fiber: The indigestible part of plant foods that plays a crucial role in digestive health, blood sugar regulation, and maintaining a feeling of fullness. There are two types of dietary fiber: soluble and insoluble, both of which are important for overall health.

Dry heat cooking: Cooking methods that use hot air or fat to transfer heat to food, such as roasting, grilling, or sautéing. These methods can help enhance flavors through browning reactions while requiring minimal added fats or oils.

E

Emulsification: The process of combining two liquids that don't normally mix, such as oil and vinegar, to create a smooth, uniform mixture. This technique is often used in making healthy salad dressings and sauces without relying on store-bought, processed alternatives.

Essential amino acids: The nine amino acids that the human body cannot produce on its own and must obtain from food sources. These are crucial for various bodily functions, including muscle building and repair. Complete proteins, such as those found in animal products, quinoa, and soy, contain all essential amino acids.

Extraction: The process of removing specific components from a food or ingredient, often used in the context of juicing or making plant-based milks. While extraction can concentrate certain nutrients, it's important to consider that some beneficial components, like fiber, may be lost in the process.

F

Fermentation: A metabolic process in which microorganisms break down sugars and starches in food, producing beneficial bacteria, enzymes, and other compounds. Fermented foods like yogurt, kefir, and sauerkraut can support gut health and enhance the bioavailability of certain nutrients.

Free radicals: Unstable molecules that can damage cells in the body, potentially leading to various health issues and accelerated aging. Antioxidants found in many fruits, vegetables, and other plant-based foods help neutralize free radicals and protect cells from damage.

Functional foods: Foods that provide health benefits beyond their basic nutritional value. Examples include foods fortified with vitamins or minerals, as well as naturally nutrient-dense foods like berries, nuts, and leafy greens that contain compounds with specific health-promoting properties.

G

Glycemic index (*GI*): A measure of how quickly a food raises blood sugar levels. Foods with a low GI are digested and absorbed more slowly, leading to a gradual rise in blood sugar, which can be beneficial for managing weight and reducing the risk of type *2* diabetes.

Grains: The edible seeds of grasses, including wheat, rice, oats, and quinoa. Whole grains contain all parts of the grain kernel and are rich in fiber, vitamins, and minerals. Incorporating a variety of whole grains into your diet can contribute to better heart health and improved digestion.

Gut microbiome: The community of microorganisms living in the digestive tract that play a crucial role in digestion, immune function, and overall health. A diverse and balanced gut microbiome can be supported through a diet rich in fiber, fermented foods, and a variety of plant-based foods.

H

Hydroponics: A method of growing plants without soil, using mineral nutrient solutions in water. Hydroponic produce can be grown year-round and may have a smaller environmental footprint compared to traditional farming methods.

Herbs: The leaves, flowers, or stems of plants used to flavor food or for medicinal purposes. Fresh herbs can add intense flavor to dishes without the need for excessive salt or fat, making them an excellent tool for healthy cooking.

Homogenization: The process of breaking down fat globules in milk to create a uniform consistency. While this process improves the texture and shelf life of milk, some argue that unhomogenized milk may have certain health benefits.

I

Infusion: The process of extracting flavors or beneficial compounds from an ingredient by steeping it in liquid. This technique can be used to create flavorful oils, teas, or broths without adding excess calories.

Insoluble fiber: A type of dietary fiber that does not dissolve in water and helps promote regular bowel movements and digestive health. Insoluble fiber is found in foods such as whole grains, nuts, and many vegetables.

Intermittent fasting: An eating pattern that cycles between periods of fasting and eating. While not directly related to cooking, understanding this concept can help in meal planning and timing for those who choose to incorporate this approach into their lifestyle.

J

Julienne: A knife cutting technique that produces long, thin strips of vegetables or fruits. This method not only creates an attractive presentation but can also help vegetables cook more quickly and evenly.

Juicing: The process of extracting juice from fruits and vegetables, often leaving behind the pulp and fiber. While juicing can provide a concentrated source of certain nutrients, it's important to balance this with whole fruits and vegetables to ensure adequate fiber intake.

Jicama: A crisp, slightly sweet root vegetable that's low in calories and high in fiber. Jicama can be eaten raw or cooked and is an excellent addition to salads, slaws, or as a crunchy snack.

K

Kefir: A fermented milk drink similar to yogurt but with a thinner consistency and more probiotic strains. Kefir is rich in beneficial bacteria and can be a valuable addition to a gut-healthy diet.

Ketogenic diet: A high-fat, low-carbohydrate diet that aims to put the body into a state of ketosis, where it burns fat for fuel instead of carbohydrates. While not universally recommended, understanding this diet can be helpful when cooking for individuals with specific dietary needs.

Kombucha: A fermented tea beverage that contains probiotics and antioxidants. Kombucha can be a healthier alternative to sugary soft drinks and may offer benefits for gut health.

L

Lacto-fermentation: A preservation method that uses beneficial bacteria to convert sugars into lactic acid, creating an environment that prevents the growth of harmful bacteria. This process is used to make foods like sauerkraut, kimchi, and pickles.

Lean protein: Protein sources that are low in saturated fat, such as chicken breast, fish, legumes, and tofu. Incorporating lean proteins into meals can help support muscle health and satiety without excessive calorie intake.

Lectin: A type of protein found in many plant foods that can interfere with the absorption of certain nutrients. While some people advocate for reducing lectin intake, these compounds are generally harmless for most individuals when foods are properly prepared and cooked.

M

Macronutrients: The three main categories of nutrients that provide energy: carbohydrates, proteins, and fats. Balancing these macronutrients in your diet is crucial for overall health and energy levels.

Maillard reaction: A chemical reaction between amino acids and sugars that occurs when food is heated, resulting in browning and the development of complex flavors. This reaction is responsible for the appealing taste and aroma of roasted vegetables, grilled meats, and baked goods.

Micronutrients: Essential vitamins and minerals required in small amounts for various bodily functions. A diverse, whole-food-based diet is the best way to ensure adequate intake of micronutrients.

N

Nutrient density: The ratio of beneficial nutrients (like vitamins, minerals, and fiber) to the calorie content of a food. Foods with high nutrient density provide substantial nutritional benefits relative to their calorie content.

Non-stick cookware: Pots and pans with a surface coating that prevents food from sticking, allowing for cooking with less oil or fat. When choosing non-stick cookware, opt for those free from harmful chemicals like PFOA and PTFE.

Nitrates/Nitrites: Compounds found naturally in some vegetables and added as preservatives to processed meats. While naturally occurring nitrates in vegetables are generally considered harmless, those added to processed meats have been linked to potential health risks when consumed in large quantities.

O

Omega-*3* fatty acids: Essential fats that play crucial roles in brain function, inflammation reduction, and heart health. Good sources include fatty fish, flaxseeds, and walnuts.

Organic: Produce and other ingredients that are grown without the use of synthetic pesticides, chemical fertilizers, or genetically modified organisms (GMOs). Organic farming practices aim to reduce environmental impact and may result in foods with higher nutrient content.

Oxidation: A chemical reaction that occurs when food is exposed to oxygen, often leading to spoilage or nutrient degradation. Proper storage techniques and the use of antioxidants can help prevent or slow down oxidation in foods.

P

Phytochemicals: Naturally occurring compounds in plants that may have health-promoting properties. Many phytochemicals act as antioxidants and may help protect against various diseases.

Probiotics: Beneficial bacteria that support gut health and overall well-being. Probiotic-rich foods include yogurt, kefir, sauerkraut, and other fermented foods.

Poaching: A gentle cooking method where food is cooked in liquid kept just below the boiling point. This technique is excellent for preparing delicate foods like fish or eggs without the need for added fats.

Q

Quinoa: A nutrient-dense pseudocereal that is a complete protein source, containing all nine essential amino acids. Quinoa is also gluten-free and rich in fiber, making it an excellent choice for various dietary needs.

Quick-pickling: A method of preserving vegetables by briefly soaking them in a vinegar-based brine. This technique can add flavor and extend the shelf life of vegetables without the lengthy fermentation process of traditional pickling.

Quenching: The process of rapidly cooling food to stop the cooking process, often by immersing it in ice water. This technique is useful for preserving the color, texture, and nutrient content of vegetables after blanching.

R

Raw food diet: A dietary approach that emphasizes consuming uncooked and unprocessed foods. While not necessarily recommended for everyone, understanding raw food preparation techniques can add variety to your healthy cooking repertoire.

Resistant starch: A type of starch that resists digestion in the small intestine and functions similarly to fiber. Foods high in resistant starch, such as cooled potatoes or green bananas, can support gut health and help regulate blood sugar levels.

Roux: A mixture of flour and fat cooked together and used to thicken sauces. In healthy cooking, alternatives like pureed vegetables or arrowroot can often be used as thickeners instead of a traditional roux.

S

Satiety: The feeling of fullness and satisfaction after eating. Understanding factors that contribute to satiety, such as protein and fiber content, can help in creating meals that keep you feeling full and satisfied.

Sous vide: A cooking method where food is sealed in airtight plastic bags and cooked in temperature-controlled water. This technique allows for precise cooking and can help retain nutrients and moisture in foods.

Sprouting: The process of germinating seeds, grains, or legumes to enhance their nutritional value and digestibility. Sprouted foods often have higher levels of certain vitamins and minerals compared to their unsprouted counterparts.

T

Tempering: Gradually raising the temperature of a cold or room-temperature ingredient by adding small amounts of a hot ingredient. This technique is useful in preventing curdling when combining ingredients with different temperatures.

Tofu: A protein-rich food made from soybeans that can be used in a variety of dishes as a meat alternative. Tofu comes in different textures and can be prepared in numerous ways to suit various recipes.

Turmeric: A spice with potent anti-inflammatory properties, often used in cooking for its vibrant color and earthy flavor. Turmeric's active compound, curcumin, is better absorbed when consumed with black pepper.

U

Umami: Often described as the fifth taste (alongside sweet, sour, salty, and bitter), umami is a savory, meaty flavor found in foods like mushrooms, tomatoes, and fermented products. Understanding umami can help in creating satisfying dishes without relying on excessive salt or fat.

Unsaturated fats: Fats that are liquid at room temperature and are generally considered heart-healthy. These include monounsaturated and polyunsaturated fats found in foods like olive oil, avocados, and fatty fish.

Ultra-processed foods: Foods that have undergone multiple processing steps and often contain additives, preservatives, and artificial ingredients. Minimizing consumption of ultra-processed foods in favor of whole, minimally processed foods is a key principle of healthy eating.

V

Vegan: A dietary approach that excludes all animal products, including meat, dairy, eggs, and honey. Understanding vegan cooking techniques and ingredient substitutions can be valuable for creating plant-based meals.

Vinaigrette: A sauce made from a mixture of oil and vinegar, often used as a salad dressing or marinade. Making your own vinaigrettes allows for control over ingredients and can be a healthier alternative to store-bought dressings.

Vitamin *B12*: An essential vitamin primarily found in animal products that plays a crucial role in nerve function and the formation of red blood cells. Those following a plant-based diet may need to consider *B12* supplementation or fortified foods.

W

Whole grains: Grains that contain all parts of the kernel, including the bran, germ, and endosperm. Whole grains are rich in fiber, vitamins, and minerals, and have been associated with various health benefits.

Water bath: A method of cooking where a container of food is placed in a larger container filled with water, allowing for gentle, even heating. This technique is often used for delicate dishes like custards or when melting chocolate.

Whey protein: A high-quality protein derived from milk during the cheese-making process. Whey protein is often used in protein powders and can be a valuable addition to smoothies or baked goods for those looking to increase their protein intake.

X

Xanthan gum: A food additive used as a thickener and stabilizer in many gluten-free recipes. While generally considered safe, some people may be sensitive to xanthan gum.

Xylitol: A sugar alcohol used as a low-calorie sweetener. Xylitol has a lower glycemic index than sugar and may have benefits for dental health, but it can cause digestive issues in some people when consumed in large amounts.

Xylose: A type of sugar found naturally in some fruits and vegetables. Xylose is sometimes used as a low-calorie sweetener and may have prebiotic properties, supporting gut health.

Y

Yeast: A single-celled microorganism used in baking and brewing. Nutritional yeast, a deactivated form of yeast, is often used as a flavor enhancer and source of *B* vitamins in vegan cooking.

Yogurt: A fermented dairy product rich in probiotics. Greek yogurt, in particular, is high in protein and can be used as a healthier substitute for sour cream or mayonnaise in many recipes.

Yield: The amount of food produced by a recipe. Understanding yield is important for meal planning and portion control in healthy cooking.

Z

Zest: The outer, colorful skin of citrus fruits that contains aromatic oils. Zest can be used to add intense flavor to dishes without additional calories or sodium.

Zinc: An essential mineral important for immune function, wound healing, and protein synthesis. Good sources of zinc include lean meats, seafood, legumes, and whole grains.

Zoodles: Noodles made from spiralized zucchini or other vegetables, often used as a low-carb alternative to pasta. Zoodles can be a creative way to increase vegetable intake in various dishes.

This comprehensive glossary serves as a valuable reference tool as you embark on your journey to master healthy cooking. By familiarizing yourself with these terms and concepts, you'll be better equipped to understand recipes, make informed food choices, and create delicious, nutritious meals. Remember, cooking is a lifelong learning process, and this glossary is just the beginning. As you continue to explore and experiment in the kitchen, you'll undoubtedly encounter new terms and techniques to add to your culinary vocabulary. Happy cooking!

Notes

1. Aune, D., et al. (2017). Fruit and vegetable intake and the risk of cardiovascular disease, total cancer and all-cause mortality—a systematic review and dose-response meta-analysis of prospective studies. International Journal of Epidemiology, 46(3), 1029-1056.
2. Bradman, A., et al. (2015). Effect of Organic Diet Intervention on Pesticide Exposures in Young Children Living in Low-Income Urban and Agricultural Communities. Environmental Health Perspectives, 123(10), 1086-1093.
3. Yuan, G. F., Sun, B., Yuan, J., & Wang, Q. M. (2009). Effects of different cooking methods on health-promoting compounds of broccoli. Journal of Zhejiang University Science B, 10(8), 580-588.
4. Andrade, J. M., Faustino, C., Garcia, C., Ladeiras, D., Reis, C. P., & Rijo, P. (2018). Rosmarinus officinalis L.: an updated review of its phytochemistry and biological activity. Future science OA, 4(4), FSO283.
5. Viegas, O., Amaro, L. F., Ferreira, I. M., & Pinho, O. (2012). Inhibitory effect of antioxidant-rich marinades on the formation of heterocyclic aromatic amines in pan-fried beef. Journal of Agricultural and Food Chemistry, 60(24), 6235-6240.
6. Smith, J. S., Ameri, F., & Gadgil, P. (2008). Effect of marinades on the formation of heterocyclic amines in grilled beef steaks. Journal of Food Science, 73(6), T100-T105.
7. Gibis, M., & Weiss, J. (2012). Antioxidant capacity and inhibitory effect of grape seed and rosemary extract in marinades on the formation of heterocyclic amines in fried beef patties. Food Chemistry, 134(2), 766-774.

8. Gibis, M. (2016). Heterocyclic Aromatic Amines in Cooked Meat Products: Causes, Formation, Occurrence, and Risk Assessment. Comprehensive Reviews in Food Science and Food Safety, 15(2), 269-302.
9. Yuan, G. F., Sun, B., Yuan, J., & Wang, Q. M. (2009). Effects of different cooking methods on health-promoting compounds of broccoli. Journal of Zhejiang University Science B, 10(8), 580-588.
10. Hewlings, S. J., & Kalman, D. S. (2017). Curcumin: A Review of Its Effects on Human Health. Foods, 6(10), 92.
11. Baardseth, P., Bjerke, F., Martinsen, B. K., & Skrede, G. (2010). Vitamin C, total phenolics and antioxidative activity in tip-cut green beans (Phaseolus vulgaris) and swede rods (Brassica napus var. napobrassica) processed by methods used in catering. Journal of the Science of Food and Agriculture, 90(7), 1245-1255.
12. Rampersaud, G. C., Pereira, M. A., Girard, B. L., Adams, J., & Metzl, J. D. (2005). Breakfast habits, nutritional status, body weight, and academic performance in children and adolescents. Journal of the American Dietetic Association, 105(5), 743-760.
13. Whitehead, A., Beck, E. J., Tosh, S., & Wolever, T. M. (2014). Cholesterol-lowering effects of oat β-glucan: a meta-analysis of randomized controlled trials. The American journal of clinical nutrition, 100(6), 1413-1421.
14. U.S. Department of Agriculture, Agricultural Research Service. FoodData Central, 2019.
15. Swanson D, Block R, Mousa SA. Omega-3 fatty acids EPA and DHA: health benefits throughout life. Adv Nutr. 2012;3(1):1-7.
16. Messina M. Soy and Health Update: Evaluation of the Clinical and Epidemiologic Literature. Nutrients. 2016;8(12):754.
17. Wyness L. The role of red meat in the diet: nutrition and health benefits. Proc Nutr Soc. 2016;75(3):227-232.
18. Réhault-Godbert S, Guyot N, Nys Y. The Golden Egg: Nutritional Value, Bioactivities, and Emerging Benefits for Human Health. Nutrients. 2019;11(3):684.

19. Sharma KD, Karki S, Thakur NS, Attri S. Chemical composition, functional properties and processing of carrot—a review. J Food Sci Technol. 2012;49(1):22-32.
20. Slavin JL, Lloyd B. Health benefits of fruits and vegetables. Adv Nutr. 2012;3(4):506-516.
21. Di Noia J. Defining Powerhouse Fruits and Vegetables: A Nutrient Density Approach. Prev Chronic Dis. 2014;11:130390.
22. Manchali S, Murthy KN, Patil BS. Crucial facts about health benefits of popular cruciferous vegetables. J Funct Foods. 2012;4(1):94-106.
23. Liu RH. Health-promoting components of fruits and vegetables in the diet. Adv Nutr. 2013;4(3):384S-392S.
24. Leidy, H. J., et al. (2015). The role of protein in weight loss and maintenance. The American Journal of Clinical Nutrition, 101(6), 1320S-1329S.
25. Hewlings, S. J., & Kalman, D. S. (2017). Curcumin: A Review of Its Effects on Human Health. Foods, 6(10), 92.
26. Allen, R. W., Schwartzman, E., Baker, W. L., Coleman, C. I., & Phung, O. J. (2013). Cinnamon use in type 2 diabetes: an updated systematic review and meta-analysis. The Annals of Family Medicine, 11(5), 452-459.
27. Mouritsen, O. G., & Styrbæk, K. (2014). Umami: Unlocking the Secrets of the Fifth Taste. Columbia University Press.
28. Young LR, Nestle M. (2002). The Contribution of Expanding Portion Sizes to the US Obesity Epidemic. American Journal of Public Health, 92(2), 246-249.
29. Wansink B, van Ittersum K. (2006). The Visual Illusions of Food: Why Plates, Bowls, and Spoons Can Bias Consumption Volume. FASEB Journal, 20(4), A618.
30. Poore, J., & Nemecek, T. (2018). Reducing food's environmental impacts through producers and consumers. Science, 360(6392), 987-992.
31. Food and Agriculture Organization of the United Nations. (2011). Global food losses and food waste – Extent, causes and prevention.
32. Springmann, M., Clark, M., Mason-D'Croz, D., et al. (2018). Options for keeping the food system within environmental limits. Nature, 562(7728), 519-525.

33. Weber, C. L., & Matthews, H. S. (2008). Food-miles and the relative climate impacts of food choices in the United States. Environmental Science & Technology, 42(10), 3508-3513.
34. Vallejo, F., Tomás-Barberán, F. A., & García-Viguera, C. (2003). Health-promoting compounds in broccoli as influenced by refrigerated transport and retail sale period. Journal of Agricultural and Food Chemistry, 51(10), 3029-3034.
35. ENERGY STAR. (2021). ENERGY STAR Product Specifications.

Biography

Dr. *A*. Romani: Indie Author and Inspirational Storyteller.

Dr. *A*. Romani is an accomplished indie author whose passion for storytelling transcends the pages of his books, inspiring and uplifting readers around the globe. With a diverse portfolio of multiple book imprints, Dr. Romani has carved a niche for himself in the literary world, where his unique voice and compelling narratives resonate deeply with audiences seeking both entertainment and enlightenment. Born with an innate curiosity and a love for creativity, Dr. Romani embarked on his literary journey early in life. His academic pursuits led him to earn a doctorate, where he honed his skills in research and communication, laying a solid foundation for his future as an indie author. This academic background not only enriched his storytelling but also equipped him with the tools to explore complex themes and characters with depth and authenticity. As an indie author, Dr. Romani embraces the freedom of self-publishing, allowing him to maintain creative control over his work and connect directly with his readers. His books span various genres each infused with his signature blend of inspiration and insight. Whether delving into fiction that reflects the human experience or crafting non-fiction that offers practical guidance, Dr. Romani's writing is characterized by its relatability and emotional resonance. Beyond his literary achievements, Dr. Romani has been deeply committed to helping others. He believes in the transformative power of stories to heal, motivate, and empower individuals. Through speaking engagements and community outreach, he shares his knowledge and experiences, encouraging others to find that special dream. All who know him will tell you that his dedication to inspiring others is evident in his interactions, where he fosters a supportive environment for creativity and personal growth. Dr. Romani's journey as an indie author is not just about publishing books; it's about creating a movement of positivity and encouragement. He understands that every story has the potential to change lives, and he strives to be a beacon of hope for those navigating their own narratives. His readers often describe his work as a source of comfort and inspiration, a testament to his ability to connect on a profound level. In a world where stories can sometimes feel fleeting, Dr. *A*. Romani stands out as a storyteller who is not only dedicated to his craft but also to the people he serves. With each new book, he continually tries to inspire, uplift, and help others, proving that the power of storytelling is limitless. As he looks to the future, Dr. Romani remains committed to his mission of making a positive impact through his writing, one story at a time.

www.ingramcontent.com/pod-product-compliance
Lightning Source LLC
LaVergne TN
LVHW062149200926
848484LV00007B/1889
* 9 7 9 8 9 9 9 0 4 3 0 0 9 *